# Reproductive Endocrinology for the MRCOG and Beyond

**Published titles in the MRCOG and Beyond series**

Antenatal Disorders for the MRCOG and Beyond *by Andrew Thomson and Ian Greer*

Fetal Medicine for the MRCOG and Beyond *by Alan Cameron, Lena Macara, Janet Brennand and Peter Milton*

Gynaecological and Obstetric Pathology for the MRCOG *by Harold Fox and C. Hilary Buckley, with a chapter on Cervical Cytology by Dulcie V. Coleman*

Gynaecological Oncology for the MRCOG and Beyond *edited by David Luesley and Nigel Acheson*

Gynaecological Urology for the MRCOG and Beyond *by Simon Jackson, Meghana Pandit and Alexandra Blackwell*

Haemorrhage and Thrombosis for the MRCOG and Beyond *edited by Anne Harper*

Intrapartum Care for the MRCOG and beyond *by Thomas F. Baskett and Sabaratnam Arulkumaran, with a chapter on Neonatal Resuscitation by John McIntyre and a chapter on Perinatal Loss by Carolyn Basak*

Management of Infertility for the MRCOG and Beyond, Second edition, *by Siladitya Bhattacharya and Mark Hamilton*

Medical Genetics for the MRCOG and Beyond *by Michael Connor*

Menopause for the MRCOG and Beyond *by Margaret Rees*

Menstrual Problems for the MRCOG *by Mary Ann Lumsden, Jane Norman and Hilary Critchley*

Neonatology for the MRCOG *by Peter Dear and Simon Newell*

Reproductive Endocrinology for the MRCOG and Beyond *edited by Michael Connor*

The MRCOG: A Guide to the Examination *by Ian Johnson et al.*

**Forthcoming titles in the series**

Early Pregnancy Issues

Epidemiology and Statistics

Molecular Medicine

# Reproductive Endocrinology for the MRCOG and Beyond

## Second Edition

**Edited by Adam Balen** MD, FRCOG
Professor of Reproductive Medicine and Surgery, Leeds Teaching
Hospitals Trust, Reproductive Medicine Unit, Clarendon Wing,
General Infirmary at Leeds, Belmont Grove, Leeds LS2 9NS

**Series Editor: Jenny Higham** MD, FRCOG, FFFP, ILTM
Consultant Obstetrician and Gynaecologist and
Head of Undergraduate Medicine, Faculty of Medicine, Imperial College
London, South Kensington Campus, Sir Alexander Fleming Building,
London SW7 2AZ

Published by the **RCOG Press**
at the Royal College of Obstetricians and Gynaecologists
27 Sussex Place, Regent's Park, London NW1 4RG

www.rcog.org.uk

Registered charity no. 213280

First published 2003; this edition published 2007

The rights of Adam Balen, Mary Birdsall, Guy Fender, Gillian Lockwood, Katherine Michelmore, Ken Ong, Margaret Rees, Madhurima Rajkhowa and John Seaton to be identified as authors of this work have been asserted by them in accordance with the Copyright, Designs and Patents Act, 1988.

ISBN 978-1-904752-19-6

*Cover illustration:*

RCOG Editor: Jane Moody
Design/typesetting: Tony Crowley

Printed by Latimer Trend & Co. Ltd, Estover Road, Plymouth PL6 7PL, UK

# Contents

# Acknowledgments

The following authors contributed to the book:

Mary Birdsall MSc(Oxon) FRANZOG
Consultant, Fertility Associates, Ascot Hospital, Greenlane Road East, Private
Bag 28910, Remuera, Auckland, New Zealand

Guy Fender MRCGP MRCOG
Consultant, Department of Obstetrics and Gynaecology,
Taunton and Somerset Hospital, Musgrove Park, Taunton, Somerset

Gillian Lockwood MA MRCOG
Medical Director, Midland Fertility Services, Centre House, Court Parade,
Aldridge WS9 8LT

Katherine F Michelmore DPhil MRCGP
Formerly Research Fellow, Nuffield Department of Epidemiology,
Oxford University, Oxford OX3 9DU

Ken Ong DPhil MRCP
Research Fellow, Department of Paediatrics, Addenbrooke's Hospital,
Cambridge CB2 2QQ

Margaret Rees DPhil FRCOG
Senior Clinical Lecturer, Nuffield Department of Obstetrics and Gynaecology,
The John Radcliffe Hospital, Headley Way, Headington, Oxford OX3 9DU

Madhurima Rajkhowa MD MRCOG
Consultant Obstetrician and Gynaecologist and Subspecialist in Reproductive
Medicine, Department of Obstetrics and Gynaecology,
Ninewells Hospital, Dundee DD1 9SY

John Seaton MRCOG
Clinical Director and Consultant, Department of Obstetrics and Gynaecology,
William Harvey Hospital, Kennington Road, Willesborough, Ashford, Kent

# Preface to the first edition

To understand endocrinology is to understand the key processes that affect normal reproductive function. A knowledge of normal endocrinology and the pathophysiology of endocrine disorders is important when dealing with disorders of reproduction. *Reproductive Endocrinology for the MRCOG and Beyond* aims to provide a comprehensive background for all gynaecologists.

Adam Balen,
*Leeds 2002*

# Preface to the second edition

It is a pleasure to have an updated version of the highly regarded first edition of *Reproductive Endocrinology for the MRCOG and Beyond* series. It is testimony to the popularity of the first edition, published in 2003, that it sold rapidly and there was immediate demand for a replacement. This version, as the first, has been compiled and updated by an undoubted leader in the field. Prof Adam Balen is a highly respected researcher and clinician – whith a Chair in Reproductive Medicine in Leeds and a considerable research track record. In recent years he has greatly enhanced our understanding with research publications concerning PCOS, ovarian function and fertility.

Reproductive endocrinology is a popular area of both special and subspecialty training and this book provides an excellent basic grounding for both. In addition, matters of development, menstruation and endocrine dysfunction are encountered by all gynaecologists and hence the broad appeal of this compact and accessible.

I hope you enjoy it.

Jenny Higham,
*Series Editor*

# Abbreviations

| | |
|---|---|
| ACE | angiotensin-converting enzyme |
| ACTH | adrenocorticotrophic hormone |
| AIS | androgen insensitivity syndrome |
| BMD | bone mineral density |
| BMI | body mass index |
| CAH | congenital adrenal hyperplasia |
| cAMP | cyclic adenosine monophosphate |
| COX | cyclooxygenase |
| CRH | corticotrophin-releasing hormone |
| CT | computed tomography |
| CVP | central venous pressure |
| D&C | dilatation and curettage |
| DHCC | dihydroxycholecalciferol |
| FSH | follicle-stimulating hormone |
| GHRH | growth hormone-releasing hormone |
| GnRH | gonadotrophin-releasing hormone |
| HBA$_1$c | serum glycosylated haemoglobin |
| hCG | human chorionic gonadotrophin |
| hCS | human chorionic somatomammotrophin |
| HDL | high-density lipoprotein |
| hMG | human menopausal gonadotrophin |
| hPGH | human placental growth hormone |
| HRT | hormone replacement therapy |
| ICSI | intracytoplasmic sperm injection |
| IDL | intermediate-density lipoprotein |
| IGF | insulin-like growth factor |
| IGFBP | insulin-like growth factor binding protein |
| IHD | ischaemic heart disease |
| IL | interleukin |
| IUS | intrauterine system |
| IVF | *in vitro* fertilisation |
| LAM | lactational amenorrhoea method |
| LDL | low-density lipoprotein |
| LH | luteinising hormone |

| | |
|---|---|
| LHRH | luteinising hormone-releasing hormone |
| MEN | multiple endocrine neoplasia |
| MRI | magnetic resonance imaging |
| Nd:YAG | neodymium: yttrium-aluminium-garnet |
| NSAID | nonsteroidal anti-inflammatory drug |
| NSAID | nonsteroidal anti-inflammatory drug |
| 17-OHP | 17-hydroxyprogesterone |
| PAI-1 | plasminogen activator inhibitor 1 |
| PAIS | partial androgen insensitivity syndrome |
| PCOS | polycystic ovary syndrome |
| $PGE_2$ | prostaglandin $E_2$ |
| PTH | parathyroid hormone |
| SHBG | sex hormone-binding globulin |
| SMR | standardised mortality rate |
| $T_3$ | triiodothyronine |
| $T_4$ | thyroxine |
| TBG | thyroid-binding globulin |
| TCRE | transcervical resection of the endometrium |
| TGF | transforming growth factor |
| TRH | thyrotropin-releasing hormone |
| TSH | thyroid-stimulating hormone |
| VEGF | vascular endothelial growth factor |
| VLDL | very-low-density lipoprotein |
| VMA | vanillylmandelic acid |

# 1 Sexual differentiation: intersex disorders

## Development of the internal and external genitalia

The development of female internal and external genitalia is largely independent of gonadal influence whereas, in the male, the testes are essential for sexual development. During early fetal life, the pronephros, mesonephros and metanephros develop in chronological order as renal excretory organs. The mesonephros and mesonephric (wolffian) ducts form the male genital tract, while in the female these regress to non-functional remnants. The paramesonephric (müllerian) ducts in the female develop into the internal reproductive organs and the upper third of the vagina.

## Origin of the ovaries and oocytes

Primordial follicles and oocytes are derived during fetal life and the oogonial stem cell line is lost before birth. In humans, at approximately four weeks of gestation the germ cells arise from the yolk sac and migrate along the hindgut to the genital ridge. The oogonia are able to move by pseudopodial amoeboid movements. Once the oogonia reach the genital ridge, they become associated with cortical cords and lose their motility. From weeks 5 through to 28 the oogonia undergo several mitotic divisions. At the same time, many oogonia are lost by atresia, some in their passage from the yolk sac and others once they have reached the gonad itself. Meiosis starts in approximately week nine and the life cycle of the oocyte is such that it undergoes only part of the first meiotic division entering meiotic arrest at the dictyate stage of prophase 1 (Figure 1.1). The final number of oocytes is therefore determined by three factors:

- the maximum number achieved by mitotic divisions
- the time at which they enter meiosis, preventing further increase in number
- the rate of atresia.

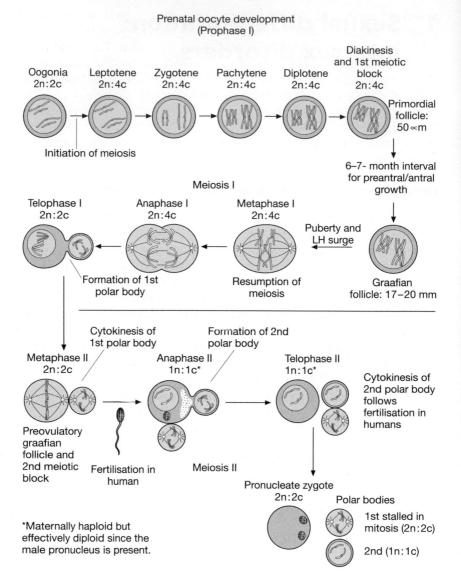

**Figure 1.1** Meiotic divisions in the oocyte; LH = luteinising hormone

The factors that affect the number of mitotic divisions and the transition from mitosis to meiosis are unknown.

From about 16 weeks of gestation, the somatic pregranulosa cells form in the genital ridge and differentiate into the granulosa cells lying on a basement membrane opposite theca cells. From about 16 weeks of gestation to six months postpartum, the oocytes secrete the zona pellucida. Thus, the primordial follicles begin to appear. The numbers of oogonia are maintained by cytokines and growth factors. The outer cortex of the ovary contains the oocytes and develops from epithelial cords within the mesenchyme of the mesonephric ridge; the medulla of the ovary regresses. The original site of the ovaries is adjacent to the kidneys before their descent into the pelvis during fetal life. The ovaries sometimes fail to complete this process and may be found anywhere from the hilum of the kidney to their final caudal position.

## Origin of the uterus and fallopian tubes

The coelomic epithelium of the upper mesonephric ridge invaginates to form the paramesonephric (müllerian) duct, which grows caudally and lateral to the mesonephric ducts before joining the genital cord and fusing with their counterpart, now ventral to the mesonephric duct. By the third month of gestation, the ends of the two paramesonephric ducts join to form the müllerian tubercle on the dorsal wall of the urogenital sinus, from which the uterine corpus and upper vagina will evolve caudally and the fallopian tubes cranially (Figure 1.2).

The mesonephric (wolffian) ducts regress, leaving vestigial structures such as the epoöphoron adjacent to the ovary and the paroöphoron, which comprise coiled tubules within the mesosalpinx that have usually disappeared by puberty. Cysts may occur by the tubal–uterine ostium (hydatids of Morgagni or appendices vesiculosae epoöphorontis) or lateral to the upper half of the vagina in remnants of the mesonephric duct (Gartner's duct cysts).

The round ligament is formed from the remains of the gubernaculum in the inguinal fold. The processus vaginalis enters the inguinal canal and usually becomes obliterated, but if patent – the canal of Nuck – may result in an inguinal hernia (Table 1.1).

## Development of external genitalia

The external genitalia are undifferentiated until 12 weeks of gestation. From eight weeks, the genital tubercle lengthens into the phallus. The urethral plate within the phallus grows towards its tip and the urethral groove develops along the caudal surface of the phallus, either side of which are the genital folds (future labia minora). Lateral to these are the genital swellings that become the labia majora.

The hymen develops from a proliferation of epithelium in the urogenital sinus. A plate of epithelium extends within the uterovaginal primordium

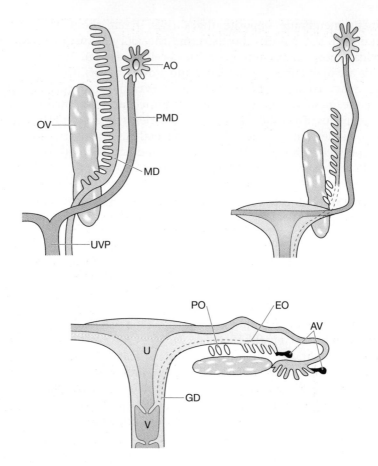

**Figure 1.2** Development of the mesonephric and paramesonephric ducts: AO, abdominal ostium; AV, appendices vesiculosae (hydatids of Morgagni); EO, epoöphoron; GD, Gartner's duct; MD, mesonephric (wolffian) duct; OV, ovary; PMD, paramesonephric duct; PO, paroöphoron; U, uterus; UVP, uterovaginal primordium; V, vagina

and is canalised in a caudocranial direction. The hymenal opening may have a variety of appearances and is occasionally imperforate.

## NEWBORN APPEARANCE

The influence of maternal hormones results in relatively large labia and a prominent clitoris at birth; the membranous fold of the hymen may project through the labia minora and the rugae of the anterior vaginal wall are also prominent and may be visible through the vaginal orifice.

**Table 1.1    Embryology of the internal and external genitalia**

| Undifferentiated | Female | Male |
|---|---|---|
| Mesonephric (wolffian) duct | Epoöphorantic (Gartner's) duct | Epididymal duct, ductus deferens, ejaculatory duct, seminal vesicle |
| Mesonephric tubules | Appendices vesiculosae | Epididymal lobules, efferent ductules, paradidymis |
| | Epoöphoron | |
| | Paroöphoron | |
| Gubernaculum | Ovarian and round ligaments | Gubernaculum testis |
| Paramesonephric (müllerian) duct | Uterus and fallopian tube | Appendix of testis, prostatic utricle |
| | Vagina: upper and lower | |
| Urogenital sinus | Urethra | Urethra |
| | Vestibule and glands | Bulbourethral glands, prostate gland |
| | Urethral and paraurethral glands | |
| Genital folds | Labia minora | Penis |
| Genital tubercle | Clitoris | Remaining penis, urethra in glans |
| Labioscrotal swellings | Labia majora | Scrotum |
| Sinus tubercle | Hymen | Seminal colliculus |
| Allantois | Urachus (median umbilical ligament) | Urachus (median umbilical ligament) |
| Dorsal cloaca | Rectum, upper anal canal | Rectum, upper anal canal |
| Ventral cloaca | Bladder, urethra | Bladder, part of prostatic urethra |

# Disorders of development of internal and external genitalia

Disorders of sexual development may result in ambiguous genitalia or anomalies of the internal genital tract and may be due to genetic defects, abnormalities of steroidogenesis and dysynchrony during organogenesis. Age of presentation will depend upon the degree of dysfunction caused. Ambiguous genitalia occur in approximately one in 30 000 newborns. The rate at which other congenital anomalies present varies depending upon the population studied and the age at which the problem is likely to be noticed. Population-based statistics are still lacking for many conditions, largely because patients present to different specialists (e.g. gynaecologists, paediatric endocrinologists, urologists) and there are rarely clear communication pathways between the different professional groups to facilitate a comprehensive service both for provision of treatment and collection of data.

Patients require sensitive care by an expert multidisciplinary group that includes gynaecologists, paediatric endocrinologists, paediatric surgeons and urologists, plastic surgeons, psychologists, specialist nurses, geneticists and urologists. A network of support should be provided both to the patient and to her parents and family. The adolescent period is a particularly sensitive time, as the individual becomes aware of her diagnosis and its impact on her sexuality, sexual function and fertility. It is particularly important to provide a seamless handover from paediatric to adult services at this time and dedicated adolescent clinics play an important role.

## MULLERIAN DUCT ABNORMALITIES

In the absence of a Y-chromosome, testis and testosterone, the wolffian duct regresses after the sixth week of embryonic life. The müllerian ducts then develop into the uterus and fallopian tubes and fuse caudally with the urogenital sinus to form the vagina. Abnormalities in the process of fusion may be either medial or vertical and result in primary amenorrhoea; complete or partial müllerian agenesis may also occur. Renal developmental abnormalities are commonly seen in association with abnormalities of the genital tract and so assessment by intravenous urography is advisable before attempting corrective surgery.

## CONGENITAL ABSENCE OF THE VAGINA

Women with Mayer–Rokitansky–Küster–Hauser syndrome (MRKH or Rokitansky syndrome) have a 46,XX genotype and a normal female phenotype with spontaneous development of secondary sexual characteristics, as ovarian tissue is present and functions normally. The müllerian ducts have failed to fuse and so there is vaginal agenesis (Figure 1.3). The incidence is about one in 5000 female births and may be associated with renal tract anomalies (15–40%) or anomalies of the skeletal system (10–20%). The external genitalia have a normal appearance but the vagina is short and blind-ending, such that either surgery or gradual dilatation is necessary to achieve a capacity appropriate for normal sexual function. Hormone treatment is not required, as ovarian estrogen output is normal. Indeed, ovulation occurs and ovarian stimulation followed by oocyte retrieval can be performed in order to achieve a 'biological' pregnancy through the services of a surrogate mother.

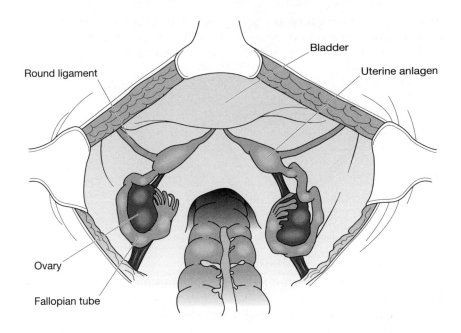

Round ligament

Bladder

Uterine anlagen

Ovary

Fallopian tube

**Figure 1.3** Appearance of pelvic cavity in case of müllerian agenesis

The vaginal dimple can vary in length from just a slight depression between the labia to 5–6 cm. Vaginal dilators, made of plastic or glass, are used first to stretch the vaginal skin and the patient is encouraged to apply pressure for 15 minutes twice daily with successive sizes of dilator. An adequately sized vagina is usually formed by six months but this may take longer and long-term use of dilators may be required, depending upon the frequency of sexual intercourse. A number of surgical approaches have been employed to create a neovagina. The Vecchetti procedure uses the same principle of progressive dilatation with the application of pressure from a plastic sphere in the vagina. The plastic sphere is attached to two wires that have been passed from the top of the vagina through to the anterior wall of the abdomen, where they are attached to a traction device that is tightened daily. Plastic surgical techniques include:

- the McIndoe vaginoplasty, in which a split skin graft is placed over a mould that has been inserted into a space created where the vagina should be (Figure 1.4)
- tissue expansion vaginoplasty, in which expansion balloons are inserted into the labia and inflated with water over a period of two weeks, in order to stretch the labial skin folds sufficiently to be used to fashion a vagina

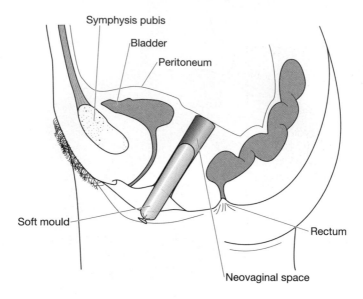

**Figure 1.4** Creation of a neovagina using a soft mould inserted into the neovaginal space

- an artificial vagina created from bowel – a technique less favoured nowadays because of problems with persistent discharge
- the Williams vaginoplasty, in which the labia are used to create a pouch – also rarely used nowadays because of problems with a poor anatomical result and an awkward angle for intercourse.

The diagnosis of Rokitansky syndrome can usually be made without the need for a laparoscopy. Sometimes, however, an ultrasound scan will reveal the presence of a uterine remnant (known as 'anlagen') that is usually small and rarely large enough to function normally. If there is active endometrial tissue within the uterine remnant, the patient may experience cyclical pain and the remnant should be excised (usually laparoscopically).

## FUSION ABNORMALITIES OF THE VAGINA

Longitudinal fusion abnormalities may lead to a complete septum, which may be associated with two complete uterine horns, with two cervices or a partial septum causing a unilateral obstruction. Excision is required both to prevent retention of uterine secretions and to permit sexual intercourse.

Transverse fusion abnormalities usually present with primary amenorrhoea and require careful assessment before surgery. The most common problem is an imperforate hymen, in which cyclical lower

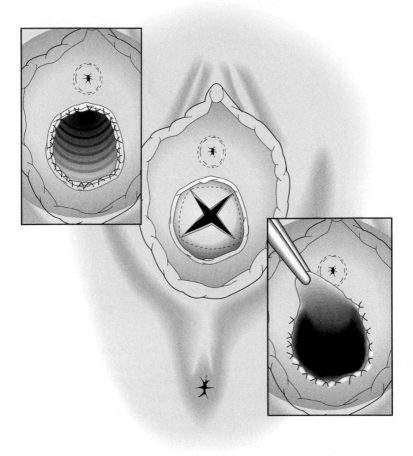

**Figure 1.5** Surgical correction of imperforate hymen: stellate incisions are made through the hymenal membrane at 2, 4, 8 and 10 o'clock positions; the individual quadrants are excised along the lateral wall of the vagina; margins of the vaginal mucosa are approximated with fine absorbable suture

abdominal pain combines with a visible haematocolpos and a bulging purple/blue hymen with menstrual secretions stretching the thin hymen (Figure 1.5). The surgery required is a simple incision that should be performed when the diagnosis is made, to prevent excessive accumulation of menstrual blood, as this may lead to a haematometra and consequent increased risk of endometriosis (secondary to retrograde menstruation). A transverse vaginal septum due to failure of fusion or canalisation between

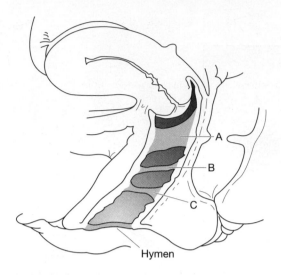

**Figure 1.6** Transverse vaginal septa; possible positions, as shown (A, B, C); 46% are high (A) and very few (14%) are low (C); sometimes there are tiny natural perforations, which permit menstrual discharge

the müllerian tubercle and sinovaginal bulb may present like an imperforate hymen but is associated with a pink bulge at the introitus as the septum is thicker than the hymen. Greater care must be taken during surgery to prevent annular constriction rings and the procedure should be performed only in dedicated centres by experienced surgeons. When there is a transverse septum, it has been found to be high in 46% of patients, in the middle of the vagina in 40% and low in the remaining 14% (Figure 1.6). It is the patients in the latter two groups who have higher pregnancy rates after surgery.

## MULLERIAN/UTERINE ANOMALIES

Uterine anomalies occur in between 3–10% of the fertile female population and can be subdivided according to the nature of the abnormality. They have been usefully classified by the American Society for Reproductive Medicine into groups (Figure 1.7):

1. Segmental agenesis or hypoplasia, which may involve the vagina, cervix, uterine corpus or fallopian tubes. Mayer–Rokitansky–Küster–Hauser syndrome is included here.
2. Unicornuate uterus, with or without a rudimentary horn, which may or may not contain endometrium and be connected to the

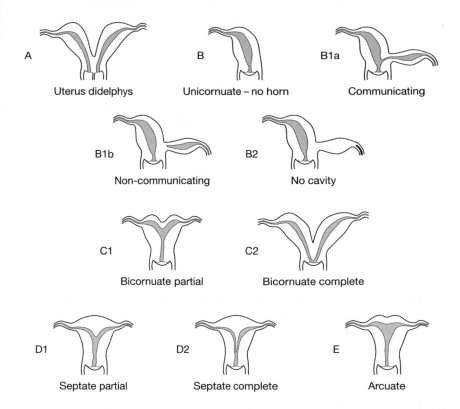

**Figure 1.7** Vertical müllerian fusion anomalies

main uterine cavity. On the affected side, the kidney and ureter are generally absent.

3. Uterus didelphys, due to partial or complete failure of lateral müllerian duct fusion leading to partial or complete duplication of the vagina, cervix and uterus.

4. Bicornuate uterus, with a single vagina and cervix and two uterine bodies, which may be completely separated or fused centrally with a partial septum.

5. Septate or arcuate uterus, with a partial or complete septum.

6. Diethylstilbestrol-related anomalies. Diethylstilbestrol was administered to prevent recurrent miscarriage in the 1950s and resulted in various anomalies of uterine development.

These anomalies are often discovered by chance during coincidental investigations for infertility. The diagnosis is made by a combination of ultrasound, magnetic resonance imaging and X-ray hysterosalpingo-graphy (the latter during the course of an infertility work-up). Women with uterine anomalies are usually asymptomatic, unless there is obstruction to menstrual flow, in which case cyclical pain may be experienced. Although infertility *per se* is rarely caused by uterine anomalies, these may be associated with endometriosis if there is retrograde menstruation secondary to obstruction. Furthermore, some women with uterine malformations may experience recurrent miscarriage.

Surgery is reserved for those cases where there is obstruction, for example the removal of a rudimentary uterine horn or excision of a vaginal septum. The excision of a uterine septum has been shown to improve pregnancy outcome and should be performed by an experienced hysteroscopist. On the other hand, metroplasty (Strassmann procedure) of the horns of a bicornuate uterus is seldom performed today, as its benefit has been questioned.

## Androgen insensitivity syndrome

Girls who are phenotypically normal but lack pubic and axillary hair in the presence of normal breast development are likely to have complete androgen insensitivity syndrome (CAIS), formerly known as testicular feminisation syndrome – a term that is no longer favoured. In this condition, the karyotype is 46,XY and, while testes are present, there is insensitivity to secreted androgens because of abnormalities in the androgen receptor. The incidence is approximately one in 60 000 'male' births and is inherited as an X-linked trait (the androgen receptor is on the short arm of the X chromosome). Anti-müllerian factors prevent the development of internal müllerian structures and the wolffian structures also fail to develop because of the insensitivity to testosterone. The external genitalia appear female. In about 10% of women, the defect is incomplete (PAIS – partial androgen insensitivity syndrome): the external genitalia may be ambiguous at birth, with labioscrotal fusion, and virilisation may sometimes occur before puberty.

After puberty, gonadal tissue should be removed to prevent malignant transformation (dysgerminoma), which occurs in about 5% of cases. Exogenous estrogen should then be prescribed: cyclical treatment is not required because the uterus is absent. The syndrome may be diagnosed in infancy if a testis is found in either the labia or an inguinal hernia, in which case both testes should be removed at this time because of the potential risk of malignancy. Some cases, however, present only at puberty, with primary amenorrhoea, and removal of abdominal/inguinal testes should then be performed.

Careful psychological assessment and counselling are necessary to provide an understanding of the gonadal dysfunction and necessity for hormone treatment. It may be helpful to describe the gonads as internal sexual organs that have been incompletely formed and are therefore prone to develop cancer if they are not removed. In general, a completely honest approach is favoured, so that the individual is provided with full information about her condition, its origins and management. It is certainly our experience that the vast majority of women want a full explanation of their condition and respond better to treatment if they are included in the decision-making processes. Women with these problems should be referred to centres where there are specialists experienced in their management, so that a comprehensive team approach can be provided.

### 5-ALPHA REDUCTASE DEFICIENCY

There are several uncommon intersex disorders that result in primary amenorrhoea and, while their management must be individualised, it will often broadly follow the above outline. Examples are male pseudohermaphroditism caused by 5-alpha reductase deficiency. In contrast to the androgen insensitivity syndrome, in these conditions there is deficient or absent breast development and yet normal or increased pubic and axillary hair; 5-alpha reductase deficiency is an autosomal recessive condition, diagnosed by the presence of under-virilisation (which may change at puberty) and an elevated testosterone-to-dihydrotestosterone ratio.

## Congenital adrenal hyperplasia

The most common cause of 'female pseudohermaphroditism' is CAH (discussed more fully in Chapter 2). Androgenisation of the female external genitalia may lead not only to clitoromegaly but also to fusion of the labioscrotal folds (Figure 1.8). There may also be a urethral fistula, which may require careful repair at the time of an introitoplasty. Clitoral reduction should be undertaken with care to preserve the neurovascular bundle and sensation (Figure 1.9). Surgery is sometimes undertaken during the neonatal period but is invariably required again during adolescence. As with all surgery for intersex disorders, the precise timing is open to debate, as is the degree to which the patient – as opposed to her parents or physicians – is involved in the decision-making process. There is evidence that delaying any surgery until adolescence results in the best outcome.

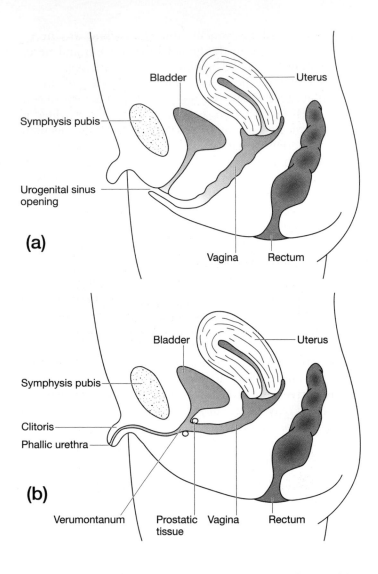

**Figure 1.8** Congenital adrenal hyperplasia: (a) mild/moderate; (b) severe

## Cloacal anomalies

Cloacal anomalies may take a variety of forms depending upon the relative contribution of gastrointestinal, genital and renal tracts. The cloaca should be divided anteriorly into the urogenital sinus and posteriorly into the rectum. Major surgery is often required during the neonatal period in order to provide anterior abdominal wall integrity and

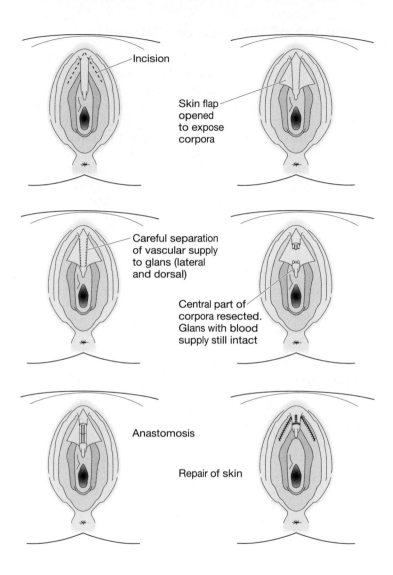

**Figure 1.9** Reduction clitoroplasty

continence of faeces and urine. Several operations may be required and the uterus and genitalia, if present, may be adversely affected such that at puberty there is obstruction to menstrual flow and also an increased rate of ovarian cyst formation, presumably due to ovarian entrapment allowing normal follicular growth and ovulation but no space for the follicle to collapse.

# Management of intersex conditions

Management of intersex conditions requires the skills of a multidisciplinary team that includes paediatric surgeons, urologists (often paediatric ands adult), plastic surgeons, endocrinologists, specialist nurses, psychologists and also the gynaecologist – whose role is to help to coordinate the transition from childhood through adolescence to womanhood and to help with issues relating to sexual function and sexual identity, endocrinology and fertility.[1] It is during the difficult time of adolescence that the patient usually first realises that there are serious problems and it is often the specialist gynaecologist who helps her to understand the diagnosis and requirements for management. The support of a skilled nurse and clinical psychologist is invaluable at this time.

# Reference

1  Houk CP, Hughes IA, Ahmed SF, Lee PA; Writing Committee for the International Intersex Consensus Conference Participants. Summary of consensus statement on intersex disorders and their management. International Intersex Consensus Conference. *Pediatrics* 2006;**118**:753–7.

# 2 Adrenal disorders

Adrenal disease is uncommon. Its diagnosis is important, however, as treatment may cure an otherwise life-threatening illness. The adrenal gland contains two endocrine organs: the adrenal medulla, which secretes catecholamines and dopamine, and the surrounding adrenal cortex, which produces steroid hormones. Catecholamines are not essential for life but they provide a mechanism for coping with stress and emergencies. The adrenal cortex, on the other hand, is essential for life. Gluco-corticoids play a role in protein and carbohydrate metabolism and mineralocorticoids are necessary for sodium balance and the maintenance of extracellular volume. The adrenal cortex also secretes sex steroids.

## The adrenal medulla

The adrenal medulla is made up of two cell types, one of which secretes adrenaline (making up 90% of the cells) and the other of which produces noradrenaline (10% of the cells). The cells contain granules and abut venous sinuses. It is unknown which cell type produces dopamine. The adrenal gland has a large blood flow.

Noradrenaline is formed by the hydroxylation and decarboxylation of tyrosine and may then be methylated to form adrenaline. The enzyme that catalyses the reaction of noradrenaline to adrenaline is only found in significant quantities in the brain and adrenal medulla. In plasma, 70% of the catecholamines are conjugated to sulphate, rendering them inactive. After adrenalectomy, noradrenaline levels are unchanged; however, adrenaline levels fall to undetectable levels. The catecholamines have a half-life of two minutes in the circulation and then are rapidly metabolised by methoxylation and oxidation to vanillylmandelic acid (VMA). Fifty percent of the secreted catecholamines appear in the urine as metanephrine and 35% as VMA. Small amounts of free catecholamines are also excreted.

### EFFECTS OF ADRENALINE AND NORADRENALINE

The catecholamines produce the 'fright or flight' response and act via alpha- and beta-adrenergic receptors. Heart rate and contractility increase,

**17**

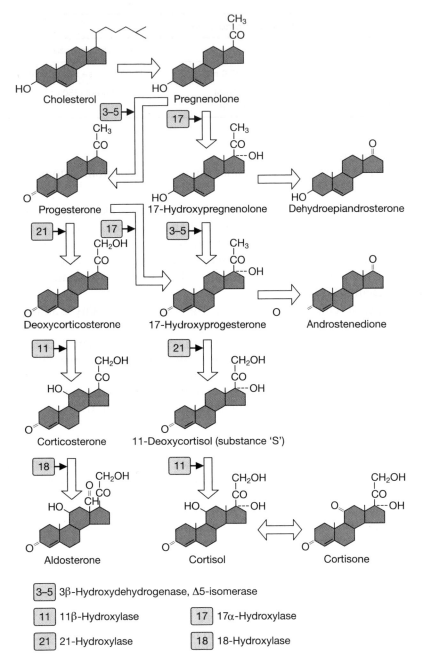

**Figure 2.1** Steroid synthetic pathway

The adrenal gland is large during fetal life, as it produces sulphate conjugates of androgens, which are then converted to estrogens by the placenta. The hormones of the adrenal cortex are derivatives of cholesterol and are of three types: $C_{21}$ steroids have a two-carbon side chain at position 17 and have mineralocorticoid and glucocorticoid actions. The term 'mineralocorticoid' refers to those steroids that are involved in sodium and potassium balance. Glucocorticoids are those concerned with glucose and protein metabolism. $C_{19}$ steroids have a keto or hydroxyl group at position 17 and have androgenic activity. $C_{18}$ steroids have a 17-hydroxy or keto group but no methyl group attached at position 10.

The adrenal cortex secretes only aldosterone, cortisol, corticosterone, dehydroepiandrosterone and androstenedione in physiologically significant amounts. Deoxycorticosterone is secreted in the same amount as aldosterone but has only 3% of its biological activity.

The major pathways for the synthesis of the adrenocortical steroids are shown in Figure 2.1. Cholesterol is taken up from low-density lipoprotein cholesterol (LDL) in the circulation. Adrenocorticotrophic hormone (ACTH) is released by the pituitary gland and binds to the receptors on the adrenal gland, which causes an increase in the uptake of cholesterol. This, in turn, increases the synthesis of pregnenolone and its derivatives. Angiotensin II binds to receptors in the zona glomerulosa, which, via a G protein, acts to increase the conversion of cholesterol to pregnenolone and thence to 18-hydroxycorticosterone. This facilitates the production of aldosterone.

ACTH is produced by the anterior pituitary gland and is a single-chain polypeptide containing 39 amino acids. The basal release of glucocorticoids and the increase in response to stress are dependent on ACTH release. Corticotrophin-releasing hormone (CRH) is a polypeptide produced by the hypothalamus and, via the portal-hypophysial vessels, stimulates the release of ACTH by the pituitary. Various neural stimuli such as emotional state via the limbic system, trauma via nociceptor pathways and the drive for circadian rhythm converge on the hypothalamus to regulate CRH secretion. Free glucocorticoids decrease ACTH secretion by the pituitary gland and CRH secretion from the hypothalamus. Chronic high glucocorticoid levels lead to diminished ACTH synthesis, which may take some time to recover. This is why high-dose exogenous steroid therapy should be reduced gradually and not withdrawn abruptly.

## HYPERFUNCTION OF THE ADRENAL CORTEX

### Congenital adrenal hyperplasia

Adrenal androgen overproduction may occur when a congenital enzymatic defect appears in one of the steroid synthetic pathways. Cortisol is the principal steroid involved in control of ACTH secretion. In CAH, due to 21-hydroxylase deficiency, the cortisol pathway is blocked and the resultant increase in ACTH secretion stimulates overproduction of adrenal androgens. Such an enzyme defect is usually inherited as an autosomal recessive trait. Severe enzyme deficiencies present with virilisation as a neonate or child (see also Chapter 1); however, partial enzyme deficiencies may not present until adolescence or early adulthood. In a female baby, CAH may present with ambiguous external genitalia, such as an enlarged clitoris or fusion of the labia: in the male, enlarged genitalia may occur. Later-onset CAH may present with virilisation in the female or precocious puberty in the male. Late-onset CAH may also present with a clinical picture similar to polycystic ovary syndrome (PCOS).

### $C_{21}$ hydroxylase deficiency

This is the most common enzymatic defect (90% of cases) and occurs in one in 14 000 births. The gene for this enzyme has been localised to the short arm of chromosome 6. In one-third of patients with 21-hydroxylase deficiency there is also an aldosterone deficiency (salt-losing variety). Diagnosis is made by measuring serum 17-hydroxyprogesterone (17-OHP), which is raised to 50–400 times above normal concentrations. In the late-onset form, serum 17-OHP concentrations are less elevated. Late-onset CAH may account for up to 2–20% of women who present with hirsutism and oligomenorrhoea, although there are racial differences and in the UK the incidence is around 2% of cases. If there is doubt about the diagnosis, an ACTH-stimulation test can be performed, with measurements of 17-OHP before and after stimulation.

The diagnosis of CAH may also be made during pregnancy, as 17-OHP and androstenedione levels are elevated in the amniotic fluid. Chorionic villus sampling using DNA probes allows the diagnosis to be made before the critical period of fetal genital differentiation (7–12 weeks). During this time, high levels of androgens cause the female fetus to have various degrees of fusion of the labial scrotal folds, clitoral enlargement and anatomical changes in the urethra and vagina (see Chapter 1). The upper reproductive tract develops normally. Androgen exposure to the female external genitalia later in pregnancy (up to 20 weeks) causes only clitoral hypertrophy. Prenatal treatment with daily dexamethasone (1.5 mg) has been shown to prevent or reduce the virilisation process. If the fetus is found to be male then therapy can be stopped. Treatment with dexamethasone has significant maternal adverse effects, including striae, hyperglycaemia, hypertension and mood changes.

### 11 beta-hydroxylase deficiency

This is the next most common enzyme deficiency and may present with virilisation as well as hypertension and hypokalaemia. The increase in blood pressure is secondary to the increase in 11-deoxycortisol and deoxycorticosterone, of which the latter is an active mineralocorticoid. The diagnosis is made by finding high levels of 17-OHP as well as deoxycorticosterone and 11-deoxycortisol. The gene for this disorder has been localised to chromosome 8 and a milder late-onset form has also been described.

## 17 alpha-hydroxylase deficiency

This rare deficiency results in a failure of production of cortisol, androgens and estradiol. It results from a variety of gene mutations on chromosome 10. The clinical presentation includes hypertension, hypokalaemia, infantile female external genitalia, absent secondary sexual characteristics at puberty and primary amenorrhoea with raised gonadotrophins. Genital ambiguity occurs in male infants. The diagnosis is made by finding increased levels of 11-deoxycorticosterone.

## 3 beta-hydroxysteroid dehydrogenase deficiency

In this enzyme deficiency, there is decreased synthesis of glucocorticoids, mineralocorticoids, androgens and estrogens. These babies are unwell at birth and frequently fail to survive. There may be mild genital ambiguity due to the enormous increase in dehydroepiandrostenedione, which at extremely high levels may be androgenic.

## 20-22-desmolase deficiency

This enzyme deficiency prevents the production of any active steroids and death is inevitable. The internal and external genitalia are female.

## Treatment of congenital adrenal hyperplasia

Glucocorticoids are required for all virilising forms of CAH, in order to replace the glucocorticoid deficit and decrease ACTH secretion. Consequently, androgen production is decreased. Suppressing ACTH also decreases the risk of developing adrenal tumours. Treatment has to be monitored carefully and overtreatment should be avoided, as excessive glucocorticoid doses may cause linear growth restriction, delay puberty and lead to cushingoid signs. In babies and infants, hydrocortisone is administered, usually twice daily. Monitoring comprises clinical evaluation of growth during childhood, bone age and pubertal development and signs of hyperandrogenism and regularity of menstrual cycle during adult life. Endocrine monitoring includes serum measurements of 17-OHP and androstenedione and 24-hour urine collections for steroid metabolites. Treatment of adults may be with hydrocortisone or the longer-acting prednisolone (usually preferred) or dexamethasone. Mineralocorticoid replacement is with fludrocortisone

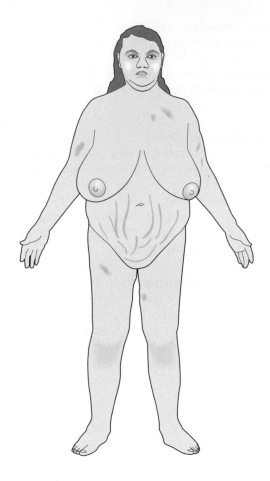

**Figure 2.2** Clinical features of Cushing's syndrome: (a) skin stretched by underlying adipose tissue, showing streaks of capillaries or striae; (b) central obesity with proximal muscle wasting; (c) 'moon face' appearance

and is monitored by serum electrolytes and plasma renin activity (which is elevated if control is suboptimal).

Surgical treatment of anatomical abnormalities should be performed in a specialist unit. Care should be taken to minimise scarring and preserve sensation. Vaginoplasty and correction of labial fusion and anomalous urethral positions is now usually delayed until adolescence. There is debate about the appropriate timing and necessity for clitoral reduction (see Chapter 1). Psychological support and counselling are required, especially during adolescence, when truculent behaviour may result in poor drug compliance and an exacerbation of the symptoms of hyperandrogenism and irregularities of the menstrual cycle (see also Chapter 1).

Pregnancy is possible if there has been adequate replacement therapy and the maintenance dose does not need to be adjusted. There will be an additional need for exogenous steroids at any time of stress, such as labour and delivery. The babies born to the mothers with these enzyme deficiencies are normal provided they have not inherited the syndrome. The neonate needs close observation for adrenal insufficiency over the first few days because steroids may cross the placenta, causing neonatal adrenal suppression.

## Cushing's syndrome

Prolonged increases in plasma glucocorticoids cause Cushing's syndrome. The glucocorticoids may be increased because of exogenous administration, glucocorticoid-producing tumours in the adrenal gland and conditions that increase ACTH secretion (Figure 2.2).

---

**CAUSES OF CUSHING'S SYNDROME**

| | |
|---|---|
| Adrenal hyperplasia | Secondary to pituitary ACTH overproduction, pituitary ACTH-producing micro- or macroadenoma (Cushing's disease), pituitary–hypothalamic dysfunction |
| | Secondary to ACTH- or CRH-producing tumour: cancer of the lung, thymus, pancreas |
| Adrenal nodular dysplasia | |
| Adrenal neoplasia | Adenoma or carcinoma |
| Exogenous causes | Glucocorticoid administration |

---

**SYMPTOMS AND SIGNS OF CUSHING'S SYNDROME**

**Symptoms**
Weakness, easy bruising, mood disorders, menstrual disorders (usually amenorrhoea)

**Signs**
Central obesity, striae, thin skin, hypertension, diabetes (20%), moon face, osteoporosis, buffalo hump, hirsutism, acne, clitoral hypertrophy, proximal myopathy

---

## Diagnosis

The first step in the diagnosis of Cushing's syndrome is to demonstrate an increase in cortisol concentrations and the next step is to determine the cause of the increased cortisol production. The dexamethasone suppression test is the most reliable initial screening test. One milligram of dexamethasone is given at 10 p.m. and a fasting plasma cortisol is taken at 8 a.m. the following morning. If the fasting cortisol is greater than 140 nmol/l, a long, low-dose dexamethasone suppression test is performed: 0.5 mg dexamethasone every six hours for 48 hours. If the plasma cortisol remains greater than 55 nmol/l and 24-hour urinary free cortisol is greater than 700 nmol/l, the diagnosis is established and the cause sought.

A high-dose dexamethasone suppression test (2 mg every six hours for two days) is then performed, together with measurement of the basal ACTH level. If basal ACTH levels are less than 1.0 pmol/l and the urinary steroids do not decrease by 40%, an adrenal tumour is likely and CT or MRI scanning arranged. If ACTH is measurable (greater than 4.5 pmol/l) and the urinary steroids decrease, an ectopic ACTH-producing tumour is unlikely and MRI of the sella turcica should be instituted.

## Treatment

Surgery is performed if an adrenal tumour is diagnosed. With bilateral hyperplasia of the adrenal gland, the ACTH- or CRH-producing pituitary tumour should also be removed. Sometimes the source of the ACTH overproduction is not apparent and there are several treatment options. In some centres, bilateral adrenalectomy is performed; in others, a surgical exploration of the pituitary via the trans-sphenoidal approach or pituitary radiotherapy is given. Medical therapy is another option: cyproheptadine or sodium valproate may decrease hypothalamic CRH release, although they are rarely used for this purpose.

## Aldosteronism

---

**SYMPTOMS AND SIGNS OF PRIMARY ALDOSTERONISM**

**Symptoms**

Headaches, muscle weakness, fatigue, polyuria, polydipsia

**Signs**

Hypertension, no oedema, cardiac arrhythmias (due to low potassium)

---

This is the syndrome of excessive production of the mineralocorticoid aldosterone. In primary aldosteronism the stimulus for increased production comes from within the adrenal gland (Conn's syndrome), and in secondary aldosteronism the stimulus is from outside. Conn's

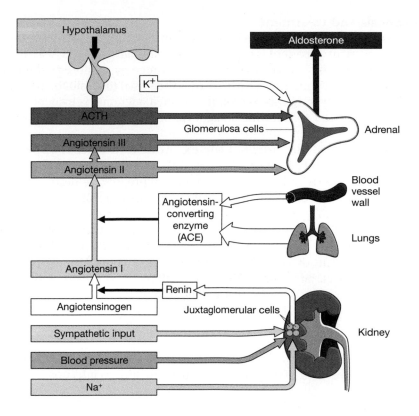

**Figure 2.3** Renin–angiotensin system: following release, renin converts angiotensinogen to angiotensin I, which is then converted to angiotensin II by the angiotensin-converting enzyme (ACE); ACTH = adrenocorticotrophic hormone

syndrome is usually caused by a small, solitary adenoma and is present in 1% of hypertensives. It is twice as common in females than males and usually presents between 30 and 50 years of age. In secondary aldosteronism, there is an appropriate increase in aldosterone secretion, secondary to activation of the renin–angiotensin system. The increase in renin is usually due to narrowing of the renal arteries.

Aldosterone causes the extracellular fluid volume to expand by increasing potassium diuresis, causing water to be retained with the osmotically active sodium ions. Prolonged potassium depletion causes muscle weakness, renal damage and metabolic alkalosis. Blood pressure increases as a consequence. Aldosterone is released in response to ACTH, potassium and through a negative feedback loop, the renin–angiotensin system (Figure 2.3).

## Diagnosis and treatment

Low serum potassium and high serum sodium, combined with hypertension in a patient not on diuretics, should lead to a search for primary aldosteronism. The diagnosis is confirmed by a failure to suppress aldosterone secretion. A CT or MRI scan is then used to locate the tumour.

Treatment is by surgical excision if a defined adenoma is evident or by spironolactone, an aldosterone antagonist, in patients where it is not.

## Hypofunction of the adrenal cortex: Addison's disease (primary adrenocortical deficiency)

Addison's disease is rare and is usually due to progressive destruction of the gland by diseases such as tuberculosis or cancer or an autoimmune process. Addison's disease may also occur in patients with other autoimmune disease such as thyroiditis, premature ovarian failure and insulin-dependent diabetes. Addison's disease may occur in HIV-positive patients as a result of rare adrenal infections or sarcomas. Ninety percent of the adrenal gland must be destroyed before clinical features become apparent. Secondary adrenocortical deficiency is more common because of the frequent use of therapeutic steroids.

## Clinical features

Presentation may be slow and insidious or present as an acute adrenal crisis, usually precipitated by some form of stress such as infection, surgery or trauma.

---

**SYMPTOMS AND SIGNS OF ADRENOCORTICAL DEFICIENCY**

**Symptoms**
Weakness, fatigability, anorexia, weight loss, nausea, vomiting
**Signs**
Mucosal and cutaneous pigmentation, hypotension, rarely hypoglycaemia and shock in acute crises

---

## Diagnosis and treatment

The diagnosis is made using ACTH stimulation tests in order to test adrenal steroid capacity.

Replacement therapy involves corticosteroids (usually prednisolone 7.5 mg daily) and mineralocorticoids (fludrocortisone 0.05–0.1 mg daily). Patients should also carry a medical alerting system. During episodes of illness or surgery the dosage of both drugs needs to be increased.

# 3 Normal puberty and adolescence

Puberty and adolescence are recognised as periods involving marked endocrine changes that regulate growth and sexual development. Normal pubertal development is known to be centrally driven and dependent upon appropriate gonadotrophin and growth hormone secretion and normal functioning of the hypothalamic–pituitary–gonadal axis. The mechanisms that control the precise timing of the onset of puberty, however, are still not clearly understood but are influenced by many factors, including general health, nutrition, exercise, genetic influences and socio-economic conditions.

## Pubertal development

Puberty represents a period of significant growth, hormonal changes and attainment of reproductive capacity. Its onset is marked by a significant increase in the amplitude of pulsatile release of gonadotrophin-releasing hormone (GnRH) by the hypothalamus. This usually occurs between the ages of eight years and 13.5 years in girls and stimulates an increase in pituitary release of luteinising hormone (LH) and follicle-stimulating hormone (FSH), which initially occurs as high-amplitude nocturnal pulses, although eventually both daytime and nocturnal pulsatile release is established. FSH and LH in turn act upon the ovary to promote follicular development and sex steroid synthesis. In the female, this period is characterised clinically by accelerated linear growth, the development of breasts and pubic hair and the eventual onset of menstruation (menarche), which occurs between the ages of 11 and 16 years in most women in the UK (Figure 3.1). Menarche is often used as a marker of pubertal development, as it is an easily identifiable event that can usually be dated with some accuracy (Figure 3.2).

In tandem with the onset of pulsatile GnRH secretion, there is an increase in the amplitude of growth hormone pulses released by the pituitary. Evidence suggests that this amplification of growth hormone secretion may be regulated by the pubertal increase in levels of both androgenic and estrogenic hormones. In addition to this action, sex steroids have been

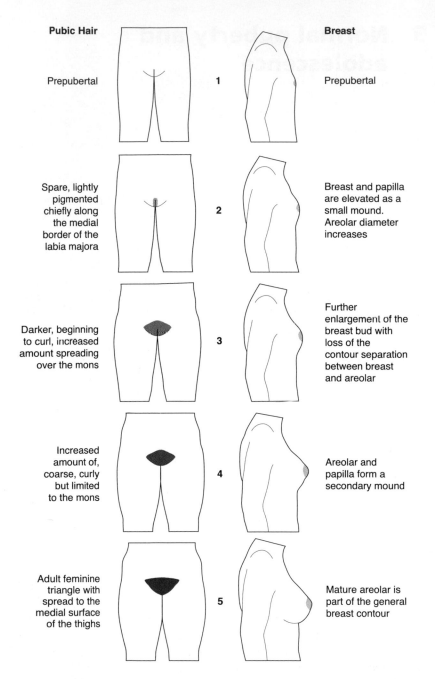

**Pubic Hair**

Prepubertal

Spare, lightly pigmented chiefly along the medial border of the labia majora

Darker, beginning to curl, increased amount spreading over the mons

Increased amount of, coarse, curly but limited to the mons

Adult feminine triangle with spread to the medial surface of the thighs

**Breast**

Prepubertal

Breast and papilla are elevated as a small mound. Areolar diameter increases

Further enlargement of the breast bud with loss of the contour separation between breast and areolar

Areolar and papilla form a secondary mound

Mature areolar is part of the general breast contour

**Figure 3.1** The Tanner stages of normal pubertal development (redrawn from Marshall and Tanner 1969, with permission)[9]

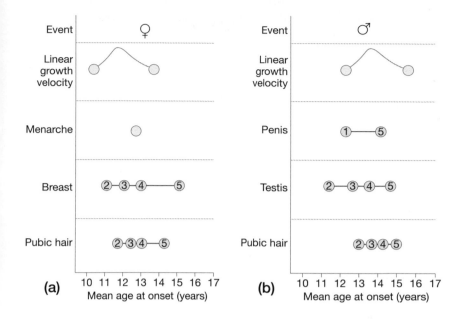

**Figure 3.2** Schematic representation of pubertal maturation in (a) females, (b) males

shown to stimulate skeletal growth directly and thus augment the role of growth hormone in promoting somatic growth and development.

Rising concentrations of growth hormone are also believed to exert some effects on circulating insulin levels, although precise mechanisms are unclear. Growth hormone induces peripheral insulin resistance, which leads to compensatory increases in insulin secretion. Increased levels of insulin during puberty may directly stimulate protein anabolism. Insulin also acts as a regulator of insulin-like growth factor 1 (IGF-1) through its effects on insulin-like growth factor-binding protein I (IGFBP-1). IGF-1 is produced by hepatic cells under the influence of growth hormone and has actions that stimulate cellular growth and maturation. IGFBP-1 competes with IGF receptors to bind IGF-1, inhibiting cellular action of IGF-1. Insulin acts to suppress production of IGFBP-1 and therefore increases circulating IGF-1 bioavailability. Insulin has also been shown to be a regulator of free sex steroids through the control of sex hormone-binding globulin (SHBG) production by the liver. Levels of SHBG decrease during puberty, and this fall parallels the rising levels of insulin. The endocrine interactions involved in normal pubertal development are represented in a simplified diagram in Figure 3.3.

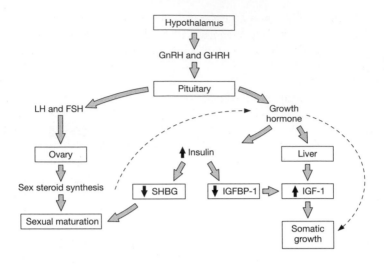

**Figure 3.3** Schematic representation of the endocrine changes that regulate pubertal development; FSH = follicle-stimulating hormone, GHRH = growth hormone-releasing hormone, GnRH = gonadotrophin-releasing hormone, IGF-1 = insulin-like growth factor 1, IGFBP-1 = insulin-like growth factor-binding protein 1, LH = luteinising hormone, SHBG = sex hormone-binding globulin

## ONSET OF PUBERTAL DEVELOPMENT

Although the endocrine changes during puberty are now better understood, the exact 'trigger' that determines onset of pulsatile GnRH release and the initiation of puberty is still unclear. The question of which factors might regulate the onset of puberty and control the rate of pubertal development has prompted extensive research. The majority of studies examining young women have used age at menarche as the key marker of sexual maturity and have attempted to elucidate which factors are involved in the timing of this event.

### Body weight and nutrition

It has long been recognised that early-maturing women have a tendency to be heavier for their heights than their later-maturing counterparts and, in contrast, that malnutrition and anorexia nervosa are associated with delayed menarche and amenorrhoea. These observed relationships between body weight and menarche led to the 'critical weight hypothesis' in which Frisch and Revelle[1] suggested that attainment of a critical body weight led to metabolic changes that in turn triggered menarche. In further work, the same investigators demonstrated that the ratio of lean body weight to fat decreased during the adolescent growth spurt in females from 5:1 to 3:1 at menarche, when the proportion of body fat was approximately 22%.[2] They suggested that adipose tissue specifically was responsible for the development and maintenance of reproductive function, through its action as an extragonadal site for the conversion of androgens to estrogens.

Although few authors will dispute that nutrition and body weight play a role in pubertal development, the 'critical weight hypothesis' for menarche has not been supported by other studies. Cameron[3] studied 36 British girls longitudinally, measuring weight and skin fold thickness at three-month intervals for the two years premenarche to two years postmenarche. They postulated that if a 'critical body fatness' was the true explanation for onset of menarche, they should expect to detect a reduction in the variability of their measurements at menarche compared with measurements taken before and after menarche and this was not demonstrated in their study. In a much larger study, Garn *et al.*[4] analysed the triceps skin fold distributions of 2251 girls collected during three national surveys in the USA. Comparing premenarchal and postmenarchal girls, they confirmed that those who had attained menarche were on average fatter than premenarchal girls. However, there was a marked overlap in skin fold thickness for both groups, and there was no evidence of a threshold level of fatness below which menarche did not occur. In another study, De Ridder *et al.*[5] performed a longitudinal assessment of 68 premenarchal schoolgirls, including pubertal staging, skin fold measurements, waist–hip ratios and blood samples for the monitoring of gonadotrophins. They did not demonstrate a relationship between body fat mass and the age at onset of puberty or age at menarche but did find that a greater body fat mass was related to a faster rate of pubertal development.

Although the above studies dispute the association of age at menarche with the achievement of a threshold weight or body fat percentage, the association of earlier maturation in heavier girls still exists. Stark *et al.*[6] reported on data from 4427 girls who were part of the National Child Development Study cohort. Data relating to birthweight, age at menarche and weights and heights measured at 7, 11 and 16 years of age were available. The authors reported that a larger proportion of girls with early menarche (before the age of 11 years) were heavier for their height at all ages when compared with those with late menarche (after 14 years). Interestingly, however, changes in relative weight in the years preceding menarche (ages 7–11 years) were not strongly associated with age at menarche, whereas being overweight at the age of seven years was much more strongly associated with an early age at menarche. Birthweight was not related to age at menarche. The authors concluded that the increase in weight for height associated with early maturation actually begins well before the onset of puberty. These findings were replicated by Cooper *et al.*,[7] who examined 1471 girls in the MRC National Survey of Health and Development. They found that girls who were heavier at the age of seven years experienced an earlier menarche; however, contrary to Stark *et al.*,[6] they found that birthweight was related to age at menarche and that girls with heavier birthweights experienced menarche at a later age.

## Exercise

Intense exercise, such as long-distance running, ballet, rowing, long-distance cycling and gymnastics, is associated with delayed menarche in young girls and with amenorrhoea in older women. These 'endurance' sports are associated with lower body weight and percentage fat. The extent to which menarche is 'delayed' has been shown to be related to the age at which participation in the sport begins and to the intensity of training. In view of the association between body weight and menarche described above, it is perhaps not surprising that girls participating in intense sporting activity experience a later age of menarche.

## Trends in menarchal age

The association between body weight and age at menarche has formed part of the basis for the explanation of the secular trend towards earlier menarche noted in the UK and other industrialised countries over the past century. It has been generally accepted that this trend has reflected improvements in nutrition, health and environmental conditions. However, a recent plateau in this trend and even a reversal in some countries have been observed that are at present unexplained. It has been suggested that this increase in menarchal age is related to changes in social conditioning in developed countries. Promotion of extremely thin women as 'ideal' role models through the media and the fashion industry has contributed to an increase in dieting in adolescent girls. Increasing participation of women in endurance sports with intense training regimens may also be a factor related to lower body weight in young girls.

## The role of insulin and leptin

These studies all indicate that pubertal development and body weight are intrinsically linked. However, the mechanism for this relationship has not been conclusively defined. Insulin has been suggested as a modulator of the tempo of pubertal development through regulation of IGFBP-1 and SHBG. States of overnutrition and obesity are associated with increased serum concentrations of insulin. Therefore, if excessive nutritional intake persists during childhood, it is possible that hyperinsulinaemia may lead to lower levels of IGFBP-1 and reduced SHBG concentrations, enhancing IGF-1 and sex steroid bioavailability. The converse would be true in states

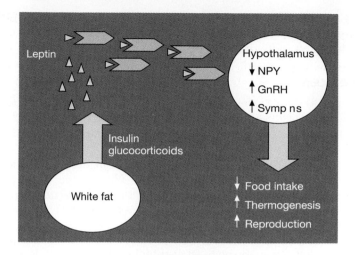

**Figure 3.4** Leptin pathway; GnRH = gonadotrophin releasing hormone; NPY = neuropeptide Y; Symp ns = sympathetic nervous system

of malnutrition, where low levels of insulin would allow for the development of increased IGFBP-1 and SHBG levels.

However, it is still unclear whether hyperinsulinaemia in childhood is a result of obesity or whether it is the cause. The role of genetic factors that may determine insulin production and obesity risk in childhood has also yet to be clearly explained. There has been much interest in the action of the recently identified hormone leptin, which is produced by adipose tissue. Serum concentrations of leptin have been shown to be related to body fat mass and it is believed that leptin exerts its action on the hypothalamus to control calorie intake, decrease thermogenesis, increase levels of serum insulin and increase pulsatility of GnRH. Through these actions, leptin may have a role in the hormonal control of pubertal development and some studies have shown that leptin levels do increase before the onset of puberty (Figure 3.4). It has been postulated that changes in circulating leptin levels may act as an initiator for the onset of puberty, and that this may explain the relationships between body fat and maturation observed by Frisch and Revelle. This hypothesis is supported by the work of Clement et al.,[8] who identified a homozygous mutation of the leptin receptor gene, which results in early-onset morbid obesity, and an absence of pubertal development in association with reduced growth hormone secretion. These findings suggest that increased leptin levels associated with gains in fat mass may signal the hypothalamus to act as an important regulator of sexual maturation. It is possible that future research may clarify the role of leptin and leptin receptors in pubertal development and may explain the variation in the timing of the onset of puberty between individuals.

## References

1  Frisch RE, Revelle R. Height and weight at menarche and a hypothesis of critical body weights and adolescent events. *Science* 1970;**169**:397–9.

2  Frisch RE. The right weight: body fat, menarche and ovulation. *Baillieres Clin Obstet Gynaecol* 1990;**4**:419–39.

3  Cameron N. Weight and skinfold variation at menarche and the critical body weight hypothesis. *Ann Hum Biol* 1976;**3**:279–82.

4  Garn SM, LaVelle M, Pilkington JJ. Comparisons of fatness in premenarcheal and postmenarcheal girls of the same age. *J Pediatr* 1983;**103**:328–31.

5  De Ridder CM, Thijssen JH, Bruning PF, Van den Brande JL, Zonderland ML, Erich WB. Body fat mass, body fat distribution, and pubertal development: a longitudinal study of physical and hormonal sexual maturation of girls. *J Clin Endocrinol Metab* 1992;**75**:442–6.

6  Stark O, Peckham CS, Moynihan C. Weight and age at menarche. *Arch Dis Child* 1989;**64**:383–7.

7  Cooper C, Kuh D, Egger P, Wadsworth M, Barker D. Childhood growth and age at menarche. *Br J Obstet Gynaecol* 1996;**103**:814–17.

8  Clement K, Vaisse C, Lahlou N, Cabrol S, Pelloux V, Cassuto D, *et al.* A mutation in the human leptin receptor gene causes obesity and pituitary dysfunction. *Nature* 1998;**392**:398–401.

9  Marshall WA, Tanner JM. Variations in the pattern of pubertal changes. *Arch Dis Child* 1969;**44**:944–54.

# 4  Abnormal puberty

## Precocious puberty

Precocious onset of puberty is defined as occurring younger than two standard deviations before the average age, which is less than eight years old in females (compared with less than nine years in males). Thus, in many girls early-onset of puberty merely represents one end of the normal distribution. However, a number of pathological conditions may prematurely activate the GnRH–LH/FSH axis, resulting in the precocious onset of puberty. Furthermore, certain physical secondary sexual features (e.g. virilisation without breast development) may occur in the absence of 'true puberty' (i.e. absent hypothalamic–pituitary activation) due to abnormal peripheral secretion of sex steroids.

---

**CAUSES OF PRECOCIOUS PUBERTY**

Gonadotrophin-dependent ('true' or 'central' precocious puberty):
- Idiopathic (family history, overweight/obese)
- Intracranial lesions (tumours, hydrocephalus, irradiation, trauma)
- Gonadotrophin-secreting tumours
- Hypothyroidism

Variants:
- Premature thelarche (and thelarche variant)
- Adrenarche

Gonadotrophin-independent:
- Congenital adrenal hyperplasia
- Sex steroid-secreting tumours (adrenal or ovarian)
- McCune–Albright syndrome
- Exogenous estrogen ingestion/administration

---

# TRUE PRECOCIOUS PUBERTY

The appearance of pubertal physical features follows the normal sequence ('consonance') beginning with breast development. The diagnosis is made by the finding of elevated basal gonadotrophin levels and, after stimulation with intravenous GnRH, the serum LH concentration is higher than FSH. It is important to consider intracranial pathology and arrange imaging if indicated.

# PREMATURE THELARCHE

Premature breast development in the absence of other signs of puberty may present at any age from infancy. Breast size may fluctuate and is often asymmetrical. Bone maturation, growth rate and final height are unaffected. The cause is unknown. The diagnosis is made by the finding of elevated FSH levels (but not LH) – both basal and post-GnRH stimulation. Ovarian ultrasound often reveals a single, large, functional cyst. It is important to monitor carefully in order to exclude the onset of true precocious puberty.

# THELARCHE VARIANT

There appears to be a wide spectrum of presentations between premature thelarche and true precocious puberty. Thus, some girls with early breast development also demonstrate increased height velocity, bone maturation and ovarian ultrasound reveals a multicystic appearance (as distinct from polycystic, see Chapter 8).

# PREMATURE ADRENARCHE

The normal onset of adrenal androgen secretion (adrenarche) occurs one to two years before the onset of puberty. Premature or 'exaggerated' adrenarche results in mild virilisation (e.g. pubic hair and acne but not clitoromegaly). The cause is unknown. The diagnosis is made by the finding of low serum gonadotrophin levels and mildly elevated adrenal androgen levels (dehydroepiandrosterone, androstenedione). It is important to exclude late-onset CAH and androgen-secreting tumours.

# CONGENITAL ADRENAL HYPERPLASIA

This is discussed in Chapter 2.

# PERIPHERAL TUMOURS

## Sex steroid-secreting tumours

Abnormal production of androgens and/or estrogens may arise from tumours of the adrenal glands (adenoma or carcinoma), ovaries (granulosa cell or theca cell neoplasia) or teratoma. Androgen-secreting tumours are usually associated with severe virilisation in young girls (less than six years old). The diagnosis is made by the finding of excessively raised circulating plasma sex hormone levels. A 24-hour urine collection for steroid profile often demonstrates excessive levels of sex steroid metabolites. Gonadotrophin levels are suppressed and alphafetoprotein levels may be raised. These tumours are often palpable and an abdominal ultrasound scan will confirm the diagnosis.

### Gonadotrophin-secreting tumours
In rare cases, a human chorionic gonadotrophin (hCG)-secreting hepatoblastoma, choriocarcinoma or dysgerminoma causes precocious puberty. Circulating levels of β-hCG are usually extremely high.

### McCune–Albright syndrome
This sporadic condition results in spontaneous activation of gonadotrophin receptors and excessive sex steroid secretion independent of normal ligand binding. It is due to a somatic activating mutation of the G protein alpha subunit, which also affects bones (polyostotic fibrous dysplasia), skin (*café au lait* spots) and potentially multiple other endocrinopathies (hyperthyroidism or hyperparathyroidism). All cells descended from the mutated embryonic cell line are affected, while cells descended from non-mutated cells develop into normal tissues. Thus, the phenotype is highly variable in physical distribution and severity. The diagnosis is made by clinical assessment, based on the presence of skin, bone and other lesions. Biopsy of affected skin may allow identification of the genetic mutation. Gonadotrophin levels are suppressed.

## MANAGEMENT OF PRECOCIOUS PUBERTY

It is important to exclude diseases that require specific therapy (e.g. CAH, cranial tumours or sex steroid-secreting tumours). Central precocious puberty may occur due to advanced hypothalamic maturation (especially if the girl's bone age is already over 11 years old).

### Inhibition of puberty
Pituitary gonadotrophin secretion can be suppressed with a GnRH agonist given by subcutaneous depot injection (either monthly or three-monthly). Circulating sex steroid levels should become undetectable and LH and FSH levels post-intravenous GnRH should return to prepubertal levels. The interval between doses of GnRH agonist may need to be shortened from four to three weeks to suppress puberty fully. Following

investigation and reassurance, however, many older girls and their parents are happy to avoid treatment.

The aims of stopping puberty are to avoid psychosocial problems arising from early sexual maturation and to prevent reduction in final adult height as a result of premature bone maturation and early epiphyseal fusion. A wrist X-ray for estimation of bone age is essential in the investigation of precocious puberty and may be used to predict final height when considering the need for treatment.

### Androgen receptor blockade

Androgen receptor blocking agents, such as cyproterone acetate, finasteride or flutamide, may be used for symptomatic treatment of excess androgen production in girls with premature adrenarche.

## Delayed puberty

Delayed puberty is defined as absence of onset of puberty by more than two standard deviations later than the average age, i.e. over 14 years in

---

**CAUSES OF DELAYED PUBERTY**

General:
- Constitutional delay of growth and puberty
- Malabsorption (e.g. coeliac disease, inflammatory bowel disease)
- Underweight (due to severe dieting/anorexia nervosa, overexercise or competitive sports)
- Other chronic disease

Gonadal failure (hypergonadotrophic hypogonadism) (see also Chapter 16):
- Turner syndrome
- Post-malignancy (following chemotherapy, local radiotherapy or surgical removal)
- Polyglandular autoimmune syndromes

Gonadotrophin deficiency:
- Congenital hypogonadotrophic hypogonadism (± anosmia)
- Hypothalamic/pituitary lesions (tumours, post-radiotherapy)
- Rare inactivating mutations of genes encoding LH, FSH or their receptors

---

females (compared with over 16 years in males). Delayed puberty may be idiopathic or familial or may result from a number of general conditions

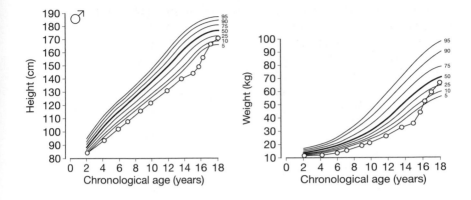

**Figure 4.1** Growth curve in constitutional delay of puberty by a) height and b) weight

leading to undernutrition. The hormone leptin is necessary for normal pubertal development and may underlie the critical weight hypothesis of Frisch (see Chapter 3). Absence of puberty may also be due to gonadal failure (elevated gonadotrophin levels) or impairment of gonadotrophin secretion. Occasionally, some girls enter puberty spontaneously but then fail to progress normally through puberty.

## CONSTITUTIONAL DELAY OF GROWTH AND PUBERTY

Rates of skeletal and sexual maturation are closely linked but vary widely between individuals and are influenced by family history and rate of early childhood weight gain. Although constitutional delay presents more commonly in males, this may merely reflect their higher level of concern. These girls are otherwise healthy. The diagnosis is made by exclusion but often can only be confirmed retrospectively following spontaneous initiation of the hypothalamic–pituitary axis (Figure 4.1).

## TURNER SYNDROME

Characteristic features of Turner syndrome may not be obvious, particularly if due to chromosomal mosaicism, and karyotype should be investigated in all girls presenting with pubertal delay. Up to 25% of girls with Turner syndrome enter puberty spontaneously but only 10% progress through puberty and only 1% develop ovulatory cycles. Thus, the chromosomal abnormality seems to result in premature ovarian exhaustion rather than a primary failure of ovarian development (see also Chapter 16). Turner syndrome is the most common cause of gonadal

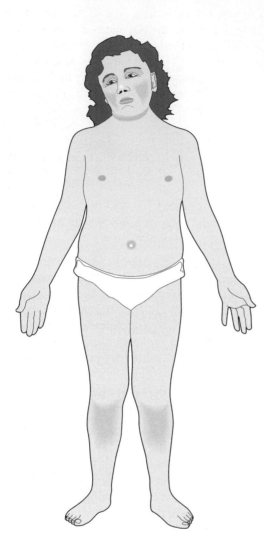

**Short stature**
less than 1.52 m
normal GH levels
poor response to GH therapy
intrauterine growth restriction

**Sexual infantilism**
dysgenetic streak-like gonads
low oestrogen; high FSH, LH

**Somatic stigmata**
FACE:
micrognathia
epicanthal folds
prominent ears
fish-like mouth
ptosis

CHEST:
widely spaced nipples

NECK:
short, webbed, low hairline

CARDIOVASCULAR:
coarctation of aorta
aortic valve disease
hypertension

RENAL:
rotation of kidney
horseshoe kidney
duplication/hydronephrosis

SKIN:
naevi
keloids
hypoplastic nails
lymphoedema

SKELETAL:
cubitus valgus
short 4th metacarpal/tarsal
high arched palate

**Figure 4.2** Features of Turner syndrome

dysgenesis. In its most severe form, the 45,XO genotype is associated with the classical features of Turner syndrome, including short stature, webbing of the neck, cubitus valgus, widely spaced nipples, cardiac and renal abnormalities and, often, autoimmune hypothyroidism (Figure 4.2). Spontaneous menstruation may occur (particularly when there is mosaicism), but premature ovarian failure usually ensues.

The clinical diagnosis is confirmed by the finding of a 45,XO karyotype (at least 30 cells should be examined due to the possibility of mosaicism). Cytogenetic analysis should also be performed looking for the presence of Y fragments, which indicate an increased risk of gonadoblastoma and the need to remove the 'streak' gonads (usually laparoscopically). Serum gonadotrophin concentrations are elevated compared with adolescents of the same age and may approach the menopausal range.

Management includes low-dose estrogen therapy to promote breast development without further disturbing linear growth. Treatment with growth hormone has also benefited some individuals. Cyclical estrogen plus progestogen may be used as maintenance therapy. A regular withdrawal bleed is essential in order to prevent endometrial hyperplasia. Spontaneous conception has been reported in patients with Turner syndrome but this is rare. However, the possibility of assisted conception and oocyte donation should be discussed at an early age.[1]

## POLYGLANDULAR AUTOIMMUNE SYNDROMES

Antiovarian antibodies are occasionally detected in both type 1 (hypoparathyroidism, Addison's disease, mucocutaneous candidiasis) and type 2 (Addison's disease, hypothyroidism, type 1 diabetes) polyglandular autoimmune syndromes. Autoimmune ovarian failure may also occur in the absence of positive antibodies due to poor sensitivity of current assays.

## CONGENITAL HYPOGONADOTROPHIC HYPOGONADISM

Congenital GnRH deficiency associated with complete or partial anosmia with or without other midline defects and mental restriction (Kallman or DeMorsier's syndrome) may be inherited in autosomal dominant, recessive or X-linked recessive patterns, suggesting that a number of mutated genes may be causative. Congenital hypogonadotrophic hypogonadism may also occur without anosmia in isolation or in panhypopituitarism. The diagnosis is made by a family history or related features of Kallman syndrome. Absent LH and FSH response to intravenous GnRH stimulation may be indistinguishable from constitutional delay of puberty, and retesting may be required after completing pubertal development with exogenous estrogen.

## MANAGEMENT OF DELAYED PUBERTY

Following exclusion of other diagnoses, many patients are happy to await spontaneous pubertal development. However, severe delay in pubertal onset may be a risk factor for decreased bone mineral density and osteoporosis. In subjects with hypergonadotrophic hypogonadism, puberty may be induced from any age. However, in Turner syndrome, delay in induction to around 14 years old may permit maximal response to growth hormone therapy.

## Pubertal development

Oral estrogen therapy should be commenced at a low dose (e.g. ethinylestradiol 2 μg daily) and gradually increased according to breast response and age, usually by 5-μg increments every six months. Oral progesterone should be added if breakthrough bleeding occurs or when ethinylestradiol dose reaches 20 μg per day. Eventually maintenance therapy is provided either with a combined oral contraceptive pill or with a conventional, cyclical postmenopausal hormone replacement preparation. As an alternative, transdermal hormone patches may be used. There is no real evidence of advantage of one preparation over another.

## Fertility

In gonadotrophin deficiency, ovulation and fertility may be achieved by ovulation induction using either pulsatile GnRH (for hypothalamic problems) or gonadotrophin therapy (for pituitary or hypothalamic disease). If the patient with hypogonadotrophic hypogonadism is particularly anxious about future fertility, a nontherapeutic trial of exogenous pulsatile GnRH administration, via a miniature portable infusion pump, confirms pituitary responsiveness. However, induction of ovulation can also be achieved, bypassing the pituitary, by direct administration of human menopausal gonadotrophin (hMG); hMG is a more suitable choice than the more recently developed recombinant FSH preparations as it also contains LH, which is necessary to stimulate estrogen biosynthesis. Pulsatile GnRH is of course more physiological and less likely to lead to multiple follicle development and hence multiple pregnancy than hMG therapy. Patients with premature ovarian failure may choose assisted conception with donated oocytes.

# Reference

1. Bondy CA, Turner Syndrome Study Group. Care of girls and women with Turner syndrome: a guideline of the Turner Syndrome Study Group. *J Clin Endocrinol Metab* 2007;**92**:10–25.

# 5  The menstrual cycle

Regular, cyclical mono-ovulation in women is achieved by a complex interaction of hormonal signals (Figure 5.1). These prevent the 'default to atresia' that is the fate of 99.98% of the approximately two million primordial follicles that exist in the ovaries of the newborn female infant. The female reproductive system functions within an integrated classical model with hypothalamic stimulation of the pituitary by a specific releasing hormone, GnRH, resulting in pituitary secretion of luteinising hormone (LH) and follicle-stimulating hormone (FSH). The structure of GnRH is common to all mammals; it is a decapeptide and its action is similar in males and females. GnRH is produced and released from a group of connected neurons in the medial basal hypothalamus, primarily within

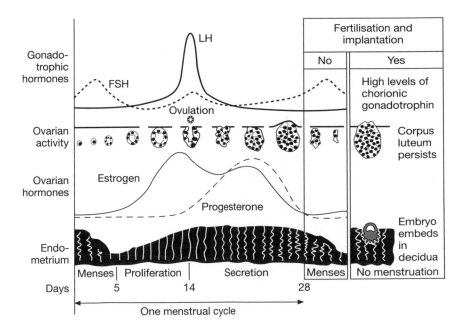

**Figure 5.1** Schematic diagram of the menstrual cycle

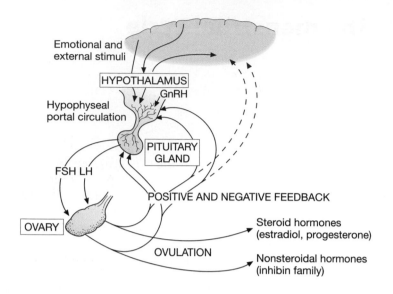

**Figure 5.2** Hypothalamic–pituitary–ovarian axis: FSH, follicle-stimulating hormone; GnRH, gonadotrophin-releasing hormone; LH, luteinising hormone

the arcuate nucleus and in the preoptic area of the ventral hypothalamus. GnRH is released by axonal transport in a pulsatile fashion into the complex capillary net of the portal system and binds to specific receptors in the plasma membrane of the anterior pituitary gonadotrophs, where it stimulates synthesis, storage and release of LH and FSH.

Physiological secretion of gonadotrophins from the pituitary requires intermittent, pulsatile GnRH secretion (Figure 5.2). The short half-life (less than three minutes) of GnRH makes it impossible to measure GnRH secretion directly in human subjects but animal studies suggest that the pulsatile pattern of LH secretion represents pulses of GnRH. Human females show a wide variation in GnRH pulse frequency, ranging from the shortest interpulse frequency of 60 minutes in the late follicular phase to approximately 216 minutes in the late luteal phase. The quality of pulsatile gonadotrophin stimulation is critical in achieving ovulation, as even minor abnormalities in the frequency or amplitude of GnRH-induced LH pulses may interfere with ovulatory function. Continuous or high-frequency pulses of GnRH or its agonist analogues result in desensitisation of the pituitary gonadotrophs and blockade of gonadal function.

The frequency and amplitude of GnRH stimulation regulate LH and FSH secretion and synthesis in a differential manner. In the early follicular phase, the LH interpulse interval is approximately 90 minutes and slowing

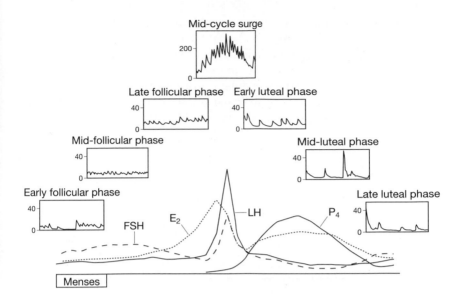

**Figure 5.3** Luteinising hormone (LH), follicle-stimulating hormone (FSH), estradiol (E$_2$) and progesterone (P$_4$) levels during the normal menstrual cycle

of the GnRH pulse generator with sleep is a unique feature of this stage of the menstrual cycle. GnRH pulse frequency increases in the midfollicular phase to every 60 minutes with a marked diminution of pulse amplitude. In the late follicular phase, GnRH pulse frequency remains at every 60 minutes while LH pulse amplitude begins a gradual increase concomitant with the rapid rise in estradiol, which sensitises the pituitary gland to GnRH (Figure 5.3).

The luteal phase is associated with a progressive decrease in the frequency of pulsatile GnRH secretion, secondary to the feedback effect of progesterone, with an interpulse interval of 100 minutes during the early luteal phase widening to four hours in the late luteal phase. The decrease in GnRH pulse frequency is associated with an increase in LH pulse amplitude.

Preantral stages of follicular growth occur independently of gonadotrophic stimulation. However, antrum formation requires stimulation by FSH, acting via its receptor in the granulosa cell surface membrane. The increment in FSH, which is required to initiate folliculogenesis, is relatively small and within the normal menstrual cycle it begins during the luteofollicular transition. The mechanisms for this increase in FSH include release from the negative feedback control of estradiol that occurs in conjunction with the demise of the corpus luteum.

A contributory mechanism is found in inhibin A, which has a suppressive effect on FSH levels during the luteal phase and is then significantly reduced as the corpus luteum fades. The luteofollicular rise in FSH occurs concomitantly with a dramatic increase in GnRH pulse frequency, suggesting that the dynamic modulation of GnRH pulse frequency that occurs between the luteal and follicular phases of the cycle may also play an important role in the luteofollicular rise in FSH.

---

**SITES OF ACTION OF HORMONES**

| | |
|---|---|
| **Endocrine** | Secreted into the circulation to have effects at distant sites |
| **Paracrine** | Secreted within a gland to have effects on other cell types within the gland |
| **Autocrine** | Factors secreted by a cell that have effects on that cell |

---

From puberty, cyclic increases in pituitary FSH secretion rescue a cohort of follicles from atresia according to the 'threshold' concept.[1] Although multiple follicles are recruited to begin preovulatory development, as the FSH concentration rises at the beginning of each cycle usually only one survives to become dominant – the follicle whose granulosa cells are most responsive to FSH. During follicular growth, FSH acts via granulosa cell FSH receptors coupled to cyclic adenosine monophosphate (cAMP)-mediated post-receptor signalling to stimulate the formation of factors that locally modulate cell proliferation and differentiation.

Autocrine factors that affect FSH-regulated granulosa cell proliferation include growth and differentiation factors such as activin and transforming growth factor (TGF) that activate serine/threonine kinase mediated post-receptor signalling.

Paracrine factors of thecal cell origin that influence FSH actions include the androgens. The granulosa cell androgen receptor that mediates the paracrine action of androgen is regulated by FSH.

Development of the dominant follicle is characterised by the secretion of increasingly large amounts of estradiol and inhibin A into the circulation, and there is evidence that the maintenance of dominance is effected by intraovarian paracrine signalling, with inhibins and activins acting as important paracrine messengers. A model has been devised by which the negative regulation of granulosa cell androgen receptor by FSH is part of the intraovarian mechanism that determines which follicle becomes dominant and hence secretes estradiol during the menstrual cycle. As follicular dominance develops, LH-stimulated thecal androgen is

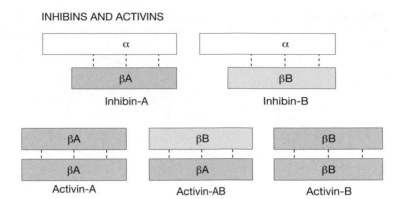

**Figure 5.4** Inhibins and activins

required as an estrogen precursor in FSH-stimulated granulosa cells. There is a role for inhibins (and insulin growth factors: IGF-1 and IGF-2) as the functional growth and differentiation factors of preovulatory follicular maturation.

Inhibin B concentrations in serum rise from early in the follicular phase to reach a peak coincident with the onset of the mid-follicular phase decline in FSH levels and then decline during the luteal phase, apart from a periovular peak that may represent release of follicular inhibin B from the rupturing follicle into the circulation.[2] By contrast, inhibin A concentrations are low in the early follicular phase, show a small midfollicular phase peak, rise rapidly with ovulation and are maximal during the midluteal phase. During the luteal–follicular transition, inhibin B concentrations rise rapidly to their mid-follicular peak, whereas inhibin A concentrations fall synchronously with estradiol and progesterone to reach a nadir at the time of the intercycle FSH peak. The different patterns of circulating inhibin A and B during the two phases of the ovarian cycle are strong evidence for their playing different physiological roles during follicular recruitment, maturation and ovulation (Figures 5.4 and 5.5).

Much experimental evidence has accrued concerning the role of activin in the female reproductive axis. Primate studies have shown that injection of recombinant human activin stimulates basal or GnRH-stimulated FSH synthesis and release and activin also regulates a variety of pituitary and ovarian hormones. During the menstrual cycle, serum activin A levels vary in a biphasic manner, with highest levels at mid-cycle during the luteofollicular transition at the specific times when FSH levels are highest and nadirs occur in the midfollicular and mid-luteal phases.

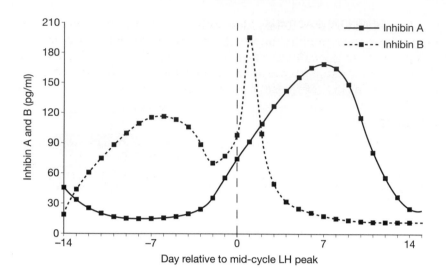

**Figure 5.5** Inhibin A and B during the menstrual cycle; LH = luteinising hormone

## Ovulation during the perimenopausal transition

An established endocrine finding associated with ageing is the rise in circulating FSH concentrations. Pituitary FSH is co-regulated by estradiol and inhibins. During the early stages of ageing, changes in estradiol that could fully account for the rise in FSH have not been consistently observed. Early follicular phase levels of inhibin B are significantly lower in older women with raised FSH than in control younger women with normal FSH. Studies of older women with normal and raised FSH show that both inhibin A (predominantly originating from the dominant follicle) and inhibin B (from the small follicles) are lower during the cycle in women with raised FSH than women with normal FSH levels. The rise in FSH without a change in estradiol is therefore due to the decline in the negative feedback effect of inhibins in the pituitary in perimenopausal women. The measurement of inhibin A (mid- to late follicular phase) and inhibin B (early follicular phase) is valuable in predicting the onset of the menopausal transition.

The complex interacting systems that regulate ovulation represent an exquisitely fine-tuned mechanism for preventing multiple ovulation while promoting regular mono-ovulation. The sensitivity of the mechanism is demonstrated by the ease with which it may become deranged, as occurs when the anorexic woman loses, or the woman with polycystic ovaries gains, a little weight. Many modern fertility treatments involving the use of pituitary desensitisation and/or the injection of exogenous gonadotrophins bypass the natural endocrine and paracrine modulators and promote multiple follicular recruitment. The current 'epidemic' of multiple births is a demonstration of the vital role of gonadotrophins in the regulation of ovulation.

## References

1  Brown JB. Pituitary control of ovarian function-concepts derived from gonadotrophin therapy. *Aust N Z J Obstet Gynaecol* 1987;**18**:47–55.
2  Groome NP, Illingworth PJ, O'Brien M, Pai R, Rodger FE, Mather JP, *et al.* Measurement of dimeric inhibin-B throughout the human menstrual cycle. *J Clin Endocrinol Metab* 1996;**81**:1401–5.

# 6  Disorders of menstruation

Disorders of menstruation are common. In a MORI national community survey in 1990, 1069 women aged 16–45 years were interviewed in their homes: 31% reported heavy periods and 38% painful periods. Of these, one-third had consulted a doctor within the past four months. The Fourth National Morbidity Survey in General Practice (1991–92) showed that for women aged 25–44 years the consultation rates for menorrhagia and dysmenorrhoea were 65 and 40 per 1000 person-years at risk, respectively, and that 5% of women aged 30–49 years consulted their GP for menor-rhagia in one year. When it comes to hospital referral, menstrual disorders are the second most common cause of all referrals for all ages and both sexes, which would appear to be a disproportionate use of health service resources by one-quarter of the population. Menorrhagia is the main presenting complaint in women referred to gynaecologists. About 73 000 hysterectomies and 10 000 endometrial ablations are performed annually in England, of which about two-thirds are undertaken for women presenting with menorrhagia.

Until recent years, by the age of 43 years one in ten women had undergone hysterectomy and 15% had undergone at least one dilatation and curettage (D&C) – the latter now considered to be obsolete, at least in the treatment of menorrhagia. The management of menorrhagia changed over the last two decades of the 20th century, with the introduction in the mid-1980s of therapeutic endoscopic endometrial destructive procedures and in 1995 of the levonorgestrel-releasing intrauterine device in the UK. The number of hysterectomies for menorrhagia has been estimated to have fallen by 36% between 1989 and 2002–03.[1,2] There also appears to be an inverse social gradient in hysterectomy, with surgery being inversely related to social class and education, especially at younger ages.

## Normal menstruation

It can be difficult for women to distinguish between normal and abnormal menstruation. The process of menstruation is poorly understood and occurs in a restricted number of species: humans and most subhuman primates. Endometrium undergoes growth, degeneration and regression before menstruation and bleeding occurs from endometrial blood vessels, especially spiral arterioles. Endometrial arterioles are unusual in that they are profusely coiled as they run through the endometrium and also change throughout the menstrual cycle. Endometrial vessels have the unique property of undergoing benign angiogenesis during each menstrual cycle; otherwise, the process of angiogenesis is restricted to neoplasia and tissue injury. Although this process is clearly under the control of ovarian steroids, endometrial endothelium lacks steroid receptors. These are present on endometrial epithelium and stromal cells, which produce angiogenic polypeptides that then act on the endothelium. The arterioles undergo profound vasoconstriction that starts 4–24 hours before menstruation and lasts until the end of menstrual bleeding. Bleeding results from relaxation of individual blood vessels and then ceases as they constrict. The myometrium contracts throughout the menstrual cycle and there is increased activity during menstruation, especially in women with primary dysmenorrhoea.

Of the pathways thought to play a major role in menstruation, the evidence for altered prostaglandin biosynthesis is the most compelling. Prostaglandins have the capacity to affect both haemostasis and myometrial contractility. High levels of prostaglandins are found in uterine tissues and menstrual blood and, furthermore, administration of prostaglandin $F_2$ alpha during the luteal phase of the cycle results in menstrual bleeding. Prostaglandin levels are further increased in women with menorrhagia and dysmenorrhoea and, clinically, inhibitors of prostaglandin biosynthesis are effective in these disorders. In menorrhagia there is additional evidence of an altered responsiveness to the vasodilator prostaglandin $E_2$. Increased concentrations of prostaglandin $E_2$ receptors are present in myometrium collected from women with excessive bleeding. In dysmenorrhoea, the leukotriene pathway allied to prostaglandins has also been implicated, in that higher levels of leukotrienes are present in endometrium of dysmenorrhoeic women. Finally, increased endometrial fibrinolysis has been implicated in menorrhagia, leading to the use of antifibrinolytic agents.

## VARIATION IN MENSTRUAL BLOOD LOSS

The amount of blood loss at each menstruation has been measured in several population studies. In several hundred women not complaining of any menstrual problems, objective measurement of menstrual blood loss shows a skewed distribution with the mean of about 35 ml and the 90th centile of 80 ml. Menstrual blood loss of greater than 80 ml is considered excessive: without treatment, such a loss leads to iron deficiency anaemia and constitutes objective menorrhagia. Blood losses of up to 1600 ml have been measured in some women. Despite variation in the total amount of blood lost, 90% is lost within the first three days of a menstrual period.

## VARIATION IN CYCLE LENGTH AND DURATION OF MENSTRUATION

Cyclical vaginal bleeding is known to occur at well-defined intervals from the menarche to the menopause. It is important that women should be informed that there is a large degree of variability in cycle length that is compatible with good health. Variability in cycle length was best evaluated in Vollman's classical study. The classical 28-day cycle happens to be the most common cycle length recorded, but only just and then in only 12.4% of cycles documented. Cycle length changes with age, forming a U-shaped curve from the menarche to the menopause. Mean cycle length drops from 35 days at the age of 12 years to a minimum of 27 days at 43 years, rising to 52 days at the age of 55 years, with an enormous range of cycle length. Clearly, there is a wide variation in normal cycle length, especially in the first few years after the menarche and in the years preceding the menopause. There are also wide variations in the duration of menstruation, which is on average five to six days.

# The abnormal menstrual cycle

## MENORRHAGIA

In objective terms, menorrhagia is a blood loss greater than 80 ml per period. Although various pathologies have been implicated in menorrhagia, in 50% of cases of objective menorrhagia no pathology is found at hysterectomy. Although 'unexplained menorrhagia' is an appropriate term, this state is often labelled less clearly as dysfunctional uterine bleeding, which implies endocrine abnormalities. It must be emphasised that most cases of menorrhagia are associated with regular ovulatory cycles and anovular cycles tend to occur soon after the menarche or close to the menopause. In ovulatory cycles, excessive menstrual loss has been ascribed to abnormal uterine levels of prostaglandins, with increased concentrations of receptors to the vasodilator prostaglandin E and elevated levels of the fibrinolytic enzyme plasminogen activator.

## ASSESSMENT OF MENSTRUAL BLOOD LOSS

A common presentation of a patient with menorrhagia is a complaint of increased menstrual loss requiring more sanitary protection or the passage of clots and flooding. Women find it difficult to assess accurately the amount of blood loss. Thus, some women who are losing several hundred millilitres consider their flow to be normal, while others losing only a few millilitres complain bitterly of menorrhagia. Furthermore, numbers of pads and tampons, as well as degree of staining, parameters often used by doctors, do not give reliable estimates. Women with true menorrhagia may not necessarily drop their haemoglobin concentration; losses of 800–1000 ml can occur without anaemia. At present, it has been estimated in hospital practice that only 40% of women complaining of menorrhagia have measured losses greater than 80 ml. Although not available routinely, objective measurement of menstrual blood loss is a valuable investigation in the assessment of heavy periods. Menstrual blood loss can easily be measured using the noninvasive alkaline haematin method, where sanitary protection devices are soaked in 5% sodium hydroxide to convert the blood to alkaline haematin, whose optical density is then measured.[3]

## CAUSES OF MENORRHAGIA

Menorrhagia may be due to systemic or pelvic pathology or to iatrogenic causes. Although disorders of haemostasis such as von Willebrand's disease and deficiencies of factors V, VII and X and idiopathic thrombocytopenic purpura are thought to increase menstrual loss, blood loss was not objectively measured in the cases originally reported. When it has been measured, platelet disorders (thrombocytopenia) rather than coagulation disorders have been implicated in menorrhagia. With regard to pelvic pathology, fibroids, endometriosis, pelvic inflammatory disease and endometrial polyps are thought to cause menorrhagia. Again there is a paucity of data with objective measurement of menstrual blood loss. The few studies where it has been measured show that these lesions are associated with objective menorrhagia in only about one-half to two-thirds of cases. Although iatrogenic causes such as intrauterine contraceptive devices have been shown to increase menstrual blood loss, there are no such data for anticoagulants.

## DIAGNOSIS OF MENORRHAGIA

History-taking and general physical and pelvic examination should enable a diagnosis to be reached. The length and interval of periods and duration of excessive bleeding, as well as any intermenstrual or postcoital bleeding, should be ascertained. The method of contraception should also be noted, since nonhormonal intrauterine contraceptive devices are associated with increased menstrual blood loss. General examination, including bimanual and pelvic examination, should be performed and a cervical smear obtained. A particular search should be made for polyps protruding through the cervical os and for enlargement or tenderness of the uterus or adnexae. A routine full blood count should be performed to check for anaemia.

The incidence of endometrial hyperplasia and carcinoma increases significantly after the age of 40 years. A prudent guideline is that biopsy is mandatory in women over that age but may be deferred in younger women unless the bleeding is severe, does not respond to treatment, is associated with intermenstrual bleeding or has occurred in an oligo/amenorrhoeic woman with polycystic ovary syndrome (see Chapter 8). However, in a woman aged over 40 years with regular periods and no intermenstrual bleeding, a trial of a prostaglandin synthetase inhibitor or an antifibrinolytic agent could be used first, since blood loss reduction tends not to occur in the presence of pathology.

# Methods of endometrial assessment

The main methods of assessment are endometrial biopsy, hysteroscopy and vaginal ultrasound.

## ENDOMETRIAL BIOPSY

### Dilatation and curettage

The classic method of obtaining endometrium is by D&C. The use of D&C has been questioned in women under the age of 40 years, since the prevalence of endometrial cancer is so low in these women. Based on estimates of endometrial cancer incidence of 0.66 per 100 000 women aged 30–34 years, it has been calculated that 3000–4000 D&C operations would have to be performed to detect one endometrial cancer in women aged under 35 years. D&C is not a risk-free procedure and it is being replaced by outpatient biopsy techniques for assessment of the endometrium. Outpatient biopsy can also be undertaken at the time of the initial consultation.

Despite having been considered a gold standard, D&C does not sample the whole of the endometrium. A study in which curettage was performed prehysterectomy found that in 60% less than one-half, and in 16% less than one-quarter, of the cavity was curetted.[4] Since D&C is essentially a blind procedure, lesions can be missed – in one study, 6% of cases (polyps, hyperplasia and carcinoma).[4] For many years, D&C was erroneously considered to be a therapeutic as well as a diagnostic procedure.

### Aspiration curettage

Vacuum or aspiration curettage was introduced in 1970. The first instrument was a 3-mm diameter stainless steel cannula with a curved tip and a wide slit on the concave surface attached to a plastic aspiration chamber and a vacuum (Vabra®, Berkeley Medevices, Berkeley, CA, USA). Since then, various types have been used with a plastic cannula (Karman®, Rocket Medical plc), which has either a 3- or 4-mm cannula. Suction can be generated either mechanically or electrically. More recently, internal piston suction devices have been devised (Pipelle®, CooperSurgical, Shelton, CT, USA; Endocell®, Wallach Surgical Devices

Inc., Orange, CT, USA). These consist of a 3-mm plastic tube with an internal piston. Its withdrawal after insertion into the uterine cavity generates suction pulling in tissue into the cannula as it is rotated. The advantage of aspiration curettage is that it avoids general anaesthesia and has fewer complications than D&C. The technical skills required for outpatient endometrial biopsy are similar to those needed to fit an intrauterine contraceptive device, and there is an argument in favour of its use in general practice after suitable training.[5]

There have been many comparative studies of the different methods that support the use of outpatient aspiration curettage. Comparisons of Vabra, Pipelle and D&C show equal accuracy. However, a comparison of Pipelle and Vabra as measured by endometrial denudation in hysterectomy specimens showed that the Pipelle sampled significantly less of the endometrial surface than the Vabra. Conversely, Pipelle is less painful than Vabra curettage. In general, any discomfort is mild and lasts for about 10–15 seconds as the cannula is passed and the biopsy taken.[6] Thus, each tool has advantages and disadvantages.

## Interpretation of endometrial biopsy reports

Proliferative and secretory changes are reported in endometrium removed from normal women. In the case of endometrial hyperplasia, the situation is more complicated because there have been several classifications over the years. The only important distinction in both prognostic and therapeutic terms is between hyperplasias, which are associated with a significant risk of progressing into an endometrial adenocarcinoma, and those devoid of such risk. It is now generally agreed that cytological atypia is the definitive feature of an endometrial hyperplasia indicative of a potentiality for malignant change. The fundamental division of endometrial hyperplasia into those with cytological atypia and those lacking this feature is therefore:

- with cytological atypia, classed as atypical hyperplasia, which can progress to carcinoma in 30% of cases, may coexist with malignant endometrium and is considered an indication for hysterectomy
- without cytological atypia, subdivided into simple and complex forms, the latter having architectural atypia where the risk of progression to malignant disease is less than 5% over 13 years, and is usually treated with progestogens (for example, medroxyprogesterone acetate 20–30 mg daily).

## HYSTEROSCOPY

The hysteroscope provides direct visualisation of the endometrial cavity and was introduced over a century ago. Flexible as well as rigid hysteroscopes are now available. It can be undertaken as an outpatient procedure. Even hysteroscopy is not 100% accurate and in rare cases adenocarcinomas are missed on initial evaluation. Although hysteroscopic evaluation of an endometrium identifies endometrial polyps and submucous fibroids more accurately than endometrial biopsy, the need for hysteroscopy in all women with abnormal uterine bleeding has not yet been confirmed. Its place is best reserved for women with persistent bleeding where endometrial biopsy is negative or the endometrium abnormally thickened on ultrasound.

## TRANSVAGINAL ULTRASOUND

This technique is increasingly being used to evaluate the endometrium. A thickened endometrium or a cavity filled with fluid is suggestive of malignancy or other pathology (hyperplasia, polyps). Premenopausally, total anteroposterior thickness (both endometrial layers) varies from 4 mm to 8 mm in the proliferative phase and peaks at 8–16 mm during the secretory phase. Detection of endometrial polyps can be enhanced by instillation of contrast medium into the uterine cavity. Whether vaginal ultrasound can replace endometrial biopsy is a matter for debate, as ultrasound does not give a histological diagnosis but is a useful adjunct.

# Initial management of menorrhagia in primary care

Women under the age of 40 years with otherwise uncomplicated regular heavy periods are extremely unlikely to have endometrial cancer or hyperplasia and referral for specialist opinion in the absence of clinically detectable pathology is unnecessary.[7] If there are no worrying signs, such as bloodstained vaginal discharge, intermenstrual or postcoital bleeding, the general practitioner can use medical therapy to try to reduce blood loss if this is what the woman wishes. The aim of therapy is to reduce blood loss to a socially convenient level at which the woman is not at risk of anaemia. In the absence of objective menstrual blood loss measurements, it must be remembered that there are two sorts of treatment failure: those with extremely heavy periods and those with a normal loss where therapy is effective only if the patient is rendered amenorrhoeic. Some women are prepared to put up with their heavy loss if it is not too debilitating or socially inconvenient and fear the adverse effects of drug therapy in the long term. Anaemia should be looked for and corrected. In women over the age of 40 years with menorrhagia, referral to a gynaecologist should be considered. However, not all women over 40 years will need referral and the general practitioner may try medical therapy first in women whose loss has been gradually increasing over the years. A sudden change in loss pattern is suggestive of pathology and needs earlier referral.

Young girls with heavy periods in the years after the menarche are extremely unlikely to have any pelvic pathology. Probably all that is required is to give reassurance by explaining to the girl and her parent that this type of menstrual upset usually settles with time. It is probably part of the maturation of the hypothalamic–pituitary–ovarian axis. General practitioners should be cautious about giving young girls hormonal treatment in the early years after the menarche because of possible long-term consequences. There are a few young girls with persistent heavy irregular periods associated with anovular cycles. In these cases, sustained unopposed estrogen levels lead to endometrial hyperplasia, which may ultimately progress in later years to carcinoma. Specialist investigation is required in these young girls to consider the need for cyclical progestogens. Rarely, menorrhagia in young girls may be the presenting feature of a coagulation defect or blood dyscrasia.

## Medical treatment of menorrhagia

First-line treatment should be medical. A wide variety of options are now available. Medical therapy is indicated when there is no obvious pelvic abnormality and the woman wishes to retain her fertility. Since menstrual loss, in the absence of pathology, does not change markedly, treatment is long-term. Thus, the drug regimen chosen must be effective, have few or mild adverse effects and be acceptable to the patient. Menorrhagia is the most common cause of iron deficiency anaemia in Western women and thus iron therapy is often indicated, as well as the options discussed below.

It is important to assess drug therapies in terms of reduction of measured menstrual blood loss, since there is poor correlation between objective and subjective assessment of blood loss. Various visual scoring techniques have been devised; however, they do not provide an objective measure. In routine clinical practice, menstrual blood loss measurements are not available; studies show that over half the women complaining of menorrhagia have a blood loss within normal limits. Here, it is the woman's perception and the effect of her menstrual flow on her quality of life that cause her to seek medical help. These factors must be taken into account when discussing treatment options. Listening to the patient's perceptions of her problem is of paramount importance in the overall management.[8]

Medical treatments for menorrhagia can be divided into two main classes: nonhormonal and hormonal. The former includes prostaglandin synthetase inhibitors and antifibrinolytics, and the latter progestogens, oral contraceptives, hormone replacement therapy, danazol, gestrinone and gonadotrophin-releasing hormone (GnRH) analogues. Nonhormonal treatment is taken during menstruation itself and should be used as the first-line therapy with either mefenamic acid or tranexamic acid. Both have been shown to be efficacious in prospective randomised trials (mefenamic acid is of additional benefit for dysmenorrhoea) and may also

| Table 6.1 | Nonhormonal treatments for menorrhagia |
|---|---|
| Treatment | Dose |
| Prostaglandin synthetase inhibitors: | |
| Mefenamic acid | 250–500 mg three times daily |
| Naproxen | 250–500 mg twice daily |
| Ibuprofen | 600 mg – 1.2 g twice daily |
| Flurbiprofen | 50–100 mg twice daily |
| Diclofenac | 50 mg two to three times daily |
| | |
| Antifibrinolytics: | |
| Tranexamic acid | 1.0–1.5 g three to four times daily |
| Ethamsylate | 500 mg four times daily |

be used together but there are no good studies of the effect of the combination. Referral for a gynaecological opinion should be considered if neither inhibitors of prostaglandin synthesis or antifibrinolytic agents are effective (Table 6.1).

## NON-HORMONAL TREATMENTS

### Prostaglandin synthetase inhibitors

Inhibitors of prostaglandin synthesis can be chemically classified into four main groups:

- salicylates (aspirin)
- indolacetic acid analogues (indometacin)
- aryl proprionic acid derivatives (naproxen, ibuprofen)
- fenamates (mefenamic acid, flufenamic acid, meclofenamic acid).

Of the four groups, the fenamates have been the most extensively studied for the treatment of menorrhagia.

The cyclooxygenase (COX) pathway with its two enzymes cyclooxygenase-1 (COX-1) and cyclooxygenase-2 (COX-2) represents one of the major routes for oxidative metabolism of arachidonic acid to prostaglandins. The demonstrated involvement of prostaglandins in the genesis of menorrhagia points to cyclooxygenase inhibitors as a potentially effective treatment. Cyclooxygenase inhibitors, commonly referred to as nonsteroidal anti-inflammatory drugs (NSAIDs), can be chemically classified into two main groups:

- COX-1 inhibitors: salicytes (aspirin), indolacetic acid analogues (indometacin), aryl proprionic acid derivates (naproxen, ibuprofen), fenamates (mefenamic acid, flufenamic acid, meclofenamic acid)
- COX-2 inhibitors: coxibs (celecoxib).

With the levonorgestrel intrauterine system (IUS), reductions of menstrual blood loss of 88% and 96% are found after 6 months and 12 months, respectively and 20% are amenorrhoeic after one year.[11,12] The levonorgestrel IUS also provides effective contraception. However, it is important to emphasise the essential difference between the levonorgestrel IUS and other intrauterine contraceptive devices, which can increase menstrual loss. The IUS is now thought to be a real alternative to surgical management for essential menorrhagia. Women also need to be counselled about irregular bleeding, which can occur in the first few months after insertion.

There are currently two progestogen-impregnated devices: the Mirena® IUS (Schering Health), which delivers 20 micrograms of LNG over 24 hours for about 5 years, and the Progestasert® IUS (Alza Pharmaceuticals, USA), which releases about 65 micrograms of progesterone over 24 hours for about 16 months. Over a three-year period, 65% of women with an LNG-IUS continue to report improved menstrual bleeding. Apart from lowering menstrual blood loss the LNG-IUS may alleviate symptoms of dysmenorrhoea and reduce the incidence of pelvic inflammatory disease. Results are comparable with endometrial resection[2,13] and it can be employed as an alternative to hysterectomy.[14] When compared with other medications and hysterectomy, the LNG-IUS is much cheaper per menstrual cycle unless it is removed before five years. The LNG-IUS showed similar efficacy and patient satisfaction at much lower costs (US$1530 for IUS versus US$4222 for hysterectomy).[14] It also preserves fertility while providing contraception and provides the progestogen for systemic hormone replacement therapy in peri-menopausal women.

### Estrogen/progestogen
The combined oral contraceptive pill is often used clinically to reduce menstrual blood loss. In general, the reduction in loss is about 50%. The mechanism of action is probably related to the induced endometrial atrophy, resulting in decreased prostaglandin synthesis and fibrinolysis. Monthly cyclical estrogen/progestogen hormone replacement therapy is also used to treat menorrhagia in perimenopausal women. Although it seems to work clinically, there have been no randomised controlled trials to date. However, open studies of three preparations have shown that measured withdrawal bleeds are no heavier than normal periods. Data on three monthly-bleed regimens are awaited.

### Danazol
Danazol is an isoxazol derivative of 17α-ethinyltestosterone that acts on the hypothalamic–pituitary–ovarian axis, as well as on the endomet-

rium, to produce atrophy. Studies have shown menstrual blood loss reductions ranging from 50% to 85%. However, the clinical use of danazol is limited by its androgenic adverse effects, which include weight gain, acne, hirsutism and rashes. It is therefore not a drug that is generally recommended.

### Gestrinone

Gestrinone is a 19-nortestosterone derivative that has antiprogestogenic, antiestrogenic and androgenic activity. In a placebo-controlled study, gestrinone was given 2.5 mg twice weekly for 12 weeks to 19 women with proven menorrhagia. Ten women became amenorrhoeic and a marked reduction in menstrual blood loss was seen in five; placebo had no effect. In three of the non-responders, submucous fibroids were found at subsequent hysterectomy. The therapy was well tolerated, since all women completed the trial. However, the androgenic adverse effects of gestrinone preclude long-term therapy.

### GnRH analogues

These agents can be used to reduce menstrual blood loss by pituitary desensitisation and subsequent inhibition of ovarian activity resulting in amenorrhoea. However, the induced hypestrogenic state with its adverse effects on bone metabolism limits its use beyond six months. When cyclical estrogen/progestogen hormone replacement therapy has been used in conjunction with GnRH analogues, median menstrual blood loss after three months of treatment in the women with objective menorrhagia was 74 ml. This treatment combination is expensive and should not be used as a first-line treatment. Specialist advice should be sought before using such regimens.

### TREATMENT FAILURES

Several options have to be considered when the patient says that the treatment has failed. First, her loss may be so excessive that, unless the treatment produces amenorrhoea, it has been insufficiently controlled. For example, with tranexamic acid where pretreatment blood loss is less than 200 ml per menstruation, 92% of women will have their blood loss reduced to less than 80 ml on therapy. However, if blood loss exceeds 250 ml, tranexamic acid is unlikely to achieve a loss within normal limits. A similar pattern would be expected with prostaglandin synthetase inhibitors. Second, she may have a pretreatment blood loss of less than 80 ml and the perceived reduction in loss on therapy is not sufficient for her. This was illustrated in a study including women with normal menstrual blood loss, in which therapy with mefenamic acid did not reduce loss and actually increased it. Lastly, the patient may have believed that estrogen exerts an effect on fibroid growth, by the stimulation of growth factors.

Uterine fibroids are usually diagnosed clinically but they may be difficult to differentiate from ovarian masses. Ultrasound is useful in this situation but, again, there may be difficulty in distinguishing between pedunculated subserous fibroids and solid ovarian tumours. If any doubt remains, patients need referral and laparoscopy and/or laparotomy may be considered.

## MANAGEMENT

The management of women with uterine fibroids depends on size and associated symptoms, as well as age and reproductive wishes. Small asymptomatic fibroids rarely require treatment but need to be monitored regularly, possibly with annual ultrasound. A concern is sarcomatous changes in fibroids, but this is now thought to be less than 0.2% and, furthermore, it may not represent change in a pre-existing fibroid but rather a *de novo* malignancy. Women with fibroids and menorrhagia are usually treated by hysterectomy. For those wishing to conserve their fertility, myomectomy may be offered.

Fibroids themselves do not appear to adversely affect fertility unless they are submucous and are distorting the endometrial cavity; in rare cases, fibroids may also block the fallopian tube(s). The advent of new endoscopic techniques means that it is possible to remove subserous and intramural fibroids by laparoscopy and submucous fibroids by hysteroscopy, and thus avoid laparotomy. Local destruction by laser or electrocoagulation is currently being evaluated.

There is a considerable demand for an alternative to surgery in the management of fibroids. Prostaglandin synthetase inhibitors are probably of limited effect in reducing heavy menstrual bleeding. The 19-norsteroids danazol and gestrinone may be effective and may indeed shrink uterine volume. A therapeutic innovation is the use of GnRH analogues to induce a temporary and reversible menopausal state. These analogues produce amenorrhoea and fibroid shrinkage. Unfortunately shrinkage is rarely complete and is not sustained after cessation of therapy. Another concern is that the bone mineral loss associated with a prolonged hypoestrogenic state limits the use of analogues to six months unless their use is combined with 'addback' continuous HRT. GnRH analogues are especially useful before hysterectomy, making the operation technically easier and reducing operative blood loss.

Uterine artery embolisation is an invasive radiological procedure that results in atrophic degeneration or transcervical expulsion of fibroids. This technique may be associated with considerable pain and hospitalisation for postoperative analgesia is often advised. Long-term follow-up studies have not been performed and it is currently felt that the procedure should only be performed in a few centres with suitably trained personnel and adequate equipment.

# Dysmenorrhoea

Dysmenorrhoea can be classified as either primary or secondary. In the former type there is no pelvic pathology, while the latter implies underlying pathology that leads to painful menstruation.

## PRIMARY DYSMENORRHOEA

In general, primary dysmenorrhoea appears 6–12 months after the menarche when ovulatory cycles have become established. The early cycles after the menarche are usually anovular and tend to be painless. Any pain usually consists of lower abdominal cramps and backache and there may be associated gastrointestinal disturbances such as diarrhoea and vomiting. Symptoms occur predominantly during the first two days of menstruation. Primary dysmenorrhoea tends not to be associated with excessive menstrual bleeding: it is rare for women to have both dysmenorrhoea and menorrhagia.

It is only in the past two decades that intrauterine pressure measurements have been performed, which demonstrated for the first time that women complaining of dysmenorrhoea were not neurotic. Primary dysmenorrhoea is associated with uterine hypercontractility, characterised by excessive amplitude and frequency of contractions and a high 'resting' tone between contractions. During contractions, endometrial blood flow is reduced and there seems to be a good correlation between minimal blood flow and maximal colicky pain, favouring the notion that ischaemia due to hypercontractility causes primary dysmenorrhoea.

It is now generally agreed that the myometrial hypercontractility pattern found in primary dysmenorrhoea is associated with increased prostaglandin production. More recently, elevated levels of leucotriene C4, D4 and E4 (substances allied to prostaglandins) have been found in endometrium collected from dysmenorrhoeic women. Increased vasopressin levels have also been implicated. Although excessive levels of prostaglandins, leucotrienes and vasopressin have been found in primary dysmenorrhoea, the primary stimulus for their production remains unknown.

## SECONDARY DYSMENORRHOEA

Secondary dysmenorrhoea is associated with pelvic pathology such as endometriosis, adenomyosis, pelvic inflammatory disease, submucous leiomyomas and endometrial polyps. The use of an intrauterine contraceptive device may also lead to dysmenorrhoea. Secondary dysmenorrhoea tends to appear several years after the menarche and the patient may complain of a change in the intensity and timing of her pain. The pain may last for the whole of the menstrual period and may be associated with discomfort before the onset of menstruation. The mechanism by which various pathologies cause pain is uncertain and, again, prostaglandins may be involved, although the evidence is less clear.

## ASSESSMENT

A full gynaecological history is an essential part of investigation. The onset of dysmenorrhoea and its relation to menstruation usually differentiate between primary and secondary dysmenorrhoea. The presence of an intrauterine contraceptive device or a history of infertility should also be noted. In young girls, one can usually assume a diagnosis of primary dysmenorrhoea and it is probably unnecessary to examine them. If the history is suggestive of secondary dysmenorrhoea, a bimanual pelvic and speculum examination should be performed. A particular search should be made for polyps protruding through the cervical os and for enlargement, tenderness or fixity of the uterus or adnexae. Referral to a gynaecologist may be necessary if pathology is suspected; investigations may include ultrasound, magnetic resonance imaging scans, hysteroscopy and laparoscopy.

## TREATMENT

The clear involvement of prostaglandins in primary dysmenorrhoea has led to the use of prostaglandin synthetase inhibitors, such as mefenamic acid, naproxen and ibuprofen, to treat the disorder, and they are effective in reducing menstrual pain in 80–90% of patients. Commencing treatment before the onset of menstruation appears to have no demonstrable advantage over starting treatment when bleeding starts. This observation is compatible with the short plasma half-life of prostaglandin synthetase inhibitors. The advantage of starting treatment at the onset of menstruation is that it prevents the patient treating herself when she is unknowingly pregnant, which would only become apparent when a period was missed.

The presence of elevated leucotriene and vasopressin levels may explain why not all women respond to prostaglandin synthetase inhibitors. The role of the various agents that affect the leucotriene pathway has not yet been fully evaluated in the treatment of primary dysmenorrhoea. Vasopressin antagonists have been examined but are not available for routine use at present. It must not be forgotten that the combined estrogen/progestogen oral contraceptive pill is a useful agent for the treatment of primary dysmenorrhoea, especially when contraception is required. The pill is effective in 80–90% of women and probably acts by reducing the capacity of the endometrium to produce prostaglandins.

Concern remains about the 10–20% of patients with primary dysmenorrhoea who fail to respond either to prostaglandin synthetase inhibitors or to oral contraceptives. Some of these women may really be suffering from secondary dysmenorrhoea with pelvic pathology, requiring appropriate investigation, but the concern has led to the examination of new agents such as leucotriene and vasopressin antagonists.

Effective treatment of secondary dysmenorrhoea must be based on a correct diagnosis since different pathologies require different therapies. In addition, the type of treatment offered must take into account the patient's age, her desire for conception, the severity of the symptoms and the extent of the disease.

# References

1. Philipp CS, Faiz A, Dowling N, Dilley A, Michaels LA, Ayers C, *et al*. Age and the prevalence of bleeding disorders in women with menorrhagia. *Obstet Gynecol* 2005;**105**:61–6.

2. Reid PC, Mukri F. Trends in number of hysterectomies performed in England for menorrhagia: examination of health episode statistics, 1989 to 2002–3. *BMJ* 2005;**330**:938–9.

3 Rees M. Role of menstrual loss measurement in management of excessive menstrual bleeding. *Br J Obstet Gynaecol* 1991;**98**:327–8.

4 Coulter A, Kelland J, Long A, O'Meara S, Sculpher M, Song F, *et al*. The management of menorrhagia. *Effective Health Care Bulletin* 1995;**9**:1–14.

5 Royal College of Obstetricians and Gynaecologists. *The Management of Menorrhagia in Secondary Care*. Evidence-based Clinical Guidelines No. 5. London: RCOG Press; 1999.

6 Rodriguez GC, Yaqub N, King ME. A comparison of the Pipelle device and the Vabra aspirator as measured by endometrial denudation in hysterectomy specimens. *Am J Obstyet Gynecol* 1993;**168**:55–9.

7 Royal College of Obstetricians and Gynaecologists. *The Initial Management of Menorrhagia*. Evidence-based Clinical Guidelines No. 1. London: RCOG Press; 1998.

8 Coulter A, Peto V, Doll H. Patients' preferences and general practitioners' decisions in the treatment of menstrual disorders. *Fam Pract* 1994;**11**:67–74.

9 Lethaby A, Augood C, Duckitt K. Nonsteroidal anti-inflammatory drugs for heavy menstrual bleeding. *Cochrane Database Syst Rev* 2002;(1):CD000400.

10 Milsom I, Andersson K, Andersch B, Rybo G. A comparison of flurbiprofen, tranexamic acid, and a levonorgestrel-releasing intrauterine contraceptive device in the treatment of idiopathic menorrhagia. *Am J Obstet Gynecol* 1991;**164**:879–83.

11 Jones K, Bourne T. The feasibility of a 'one stop' ultrasound-based clinic for the diagnosis and management of abnormal uterine bleeding. *Ultrasound Obstet Gynecol* 2001;**17**:517–21.

12 Lethaby AE, Cooke I, Rees M. Progesterone/progestogen releasing intrauterine systems versus either placebo or any other medication for heavy menstrual bleeding. *Cochrane Database Syst Rev* 2000;(2):CD002126.

13 Rauramo I, Elo I, Istre O. Long-term treatment of menorrhagia with levonorgestrel intrauterine system versus endometrial resection. *Obstet Gynecol* 2004;**104**:1314–21.

14 Hurskainen R, Teperi J, Rissanen P, Aalto AM, Grenman S, Kivela A, *et al.* Quality of life and cost-effectiveness of levonorgestrel-releasing intrauterine system versus hysterectomy for treatment of menorrhagia: a randomised trial. *Lancet* 2001;**357**:273–7.

# 7 Amenorrhoea

Amenorrhoea is the absence of menstruation, either temporary or permanent. It may occur as a normal physiological condition, before puberty and during pregnancy, lactation or the menopause, or it may be a feature of a systemic or gynaecological disorder.

## Primary amenorrhoea

The failure to menstruate by the age of 16 years in the presence of normal secondary sexual development or by 14 years in the absence of secondary sexual characteristics warrants investigation. This distinction helps to differentiate reproductive tract anomalies from gonadal quiescence and gonadal failure (Chapter 4). Primary amenorrhoea may be a result of congenital abnormalities in the development of ovaries, genital tract or external genitalia or of a disturbance of the normal endocrinological events of puberty. Most of the causes of secondary amenorrhoea can also cause primary amenorrhoea if they occur before the menarche. Delayed puberty is often constitutional but it is important to exclude primary ovarian failure and hypothalamic or pituitary dysfunction. Overall it is estimated that endocrine disorders account for approximately 40% of the causes of primary amenorrhoea, the remaining 60% having developmental abnormalities.

For causes of primary amenorrhoea other than those described under the classification of secondary amenorrhoea, see Chapter 1 for congenital developmental anomalies and Chapter 4 for endocrinological disturbances of puberty.

## Secondary amenorrhoea

Cessation of menstruation for six consecutive months in a woman who has previously had regular periods is the usual criterion for investigation. Women with secondary amenorrhoea must have had a patent lower genital tract, an endometrium that is responsive to ovarian hormone stimulation and ovaries that have responded to pituitary gonadotrophins.

## Examination and investigation of amenorrhoea

A thorough history and a careful examination of stature and body form, secondary sexual development and external genitalia should always be carried out before further investigations are instigated. A history of secondary amenorrhoea may be misleading, as the 'periods' may have been the result of exogenous hormone administration. In most cases, however, a history of secondary amenorrhoea excludes congenital abnormalities. A family history of fertility problems, autoimmune disorders or premature menopause may also give clues to the aetiology.

A bimanual examination is inappropriate in a young woman who has never been sexually active. Examination of the external genitalia of an adolescent should be undertaken in the presence of the patient's mother. Furthermore, it may be more appropriate to defer any such examination from the first consultation in order to gain an adolescent woman's confidence for future management. A transabdominal ultrasound examination of the pelvis is an excellent noninvasive method of obtaining valuable information in these patients. However, examination under anaesthetic is sometimes indicated, particularly in intersex cases.

On establishing that the internal and external genitalia are normally developed, it is important to exclude pregnancy in women of any age. Measurement of height and weight should be carried out in order to calculate a patient's body mass index (BMI). The normal range is 20–25 kg/m$^2$ and a value above or below this range may suggest a diagnosis of weight-related amenorrhoea (a term that is usually applied to underweight women).

A baseline assessment in all women should include measurement of serum prolactin and gonadotrophin concentration and an assessment of thyroid function. Prolactin levels may be elevated in response to a number of conditions, including stress, a recent breast examination or even a blood test. However, the elevation is usually moderate and transient. A more permanent, but still moderate elevation (greater than 700 iu) is associated with hypothyroidism and is also a finding in some women with polycystic ovary syndrome (PCOS), where prolactin levels up to 2000 iu/l have been reported. PCOS may also result in amenorrhoea, which can therefore create diagnostic difficulties for those women with hyperprolactinaemia and polycystic ovaries. Amenorrhoea in women with PCOS is secondary to acyclical ovarian activity and continuous estrogen production. A positive response to a progestogen challenge test, which induces a withdrawal bleed, will distinguish women with PCOS-related hyperprolactinaemia from those with polycystic ovaries and unrelated hyperprolactinaemia, because the latter causes estrogen deficiency and therefore failure to respond to the progestogen challenge (a pelvic ultrasound assessment of ovarian morphology and endometrial thickness will also provide the answer).

A serum prolactin concentration of greater than 1500 iu/l warrants further investigation. CT or MRI of the pituitary fossa may be used to exclude a hypothalamic tumour, a nonfunctioning pituitary tumour compressing the hypothalamus (e.g. craniopharyngioma) or a prolactinoma. Serum prolactin concentrations greater than 5000 iu/l are usually associated with a macroprolactinoma, which by definition is greater than 1 cm in diameter.

Serum measurements of estradiol are unhelpful as they vary considerably, even in a woman with amenorrhoea. If the woman is well estrogenised, the endometrium will be shed on withdrawal of an exogenous progestogen preparation (see above).

Serum gonadotrophin measurements help to distinguish between cases of hypothalamic or pituitary failure and gonadal failure. Elevated gonadotrophin concentrations indicate a failure of negative feedback as a result of primary ovarian failure. A serum FSH concentration of greater than 15 iu/l that is not associated with a preovulatory surge suggests impending ovarian failure. FSH levels of greater than 40 iu/l are suggestive of irreversible ovarian failure. The exact values vary according to individual assays, and so local reference ranges should be checked.

An elevated LH concentration, when associated with a raised FSH concentration, is indicative of ovarian failure. However, if LH is elevated alone (and is not attributable to the preovulatory LH surge) this suggests PCOS, which may be confirmed by a pelvic ultrasound scan (see Chapter 8). Rarely, an elevated LH concentration in a phenotypic female may be due to androgen insensitivity syndrome (AIS, previously known as testicular feminisation syndrome).

Failure at the level of the hypothalamus or pituitary is reflected by abnormally low levels of serum gonadotrophin concentrations and gives rise to hypogonadotrophic hypogonadism. Kallman syndrome is the clinical finding of hyposmia and/or colour blindness associated with hypogonadotrophic hypogonadism. It is difficult to distinguish between hypothalamic and pituitary aetiology, as both respond to stimulation with gonadotrophin-releasing hormone (GnRH). A skull X-ray is rarely performed nowadays, as much more information is provided by CT or MRI.

Karyotyping of women with primary amenorrhoea or those under 30 years with gonadotrophin levels compatible with premature ovarian failure should be performed as some chromosomal abnormalities (e.g. Turner syndrome) may be associated with premature ovarian failure. An autoantibody screen should also be undertaken in women with a premature menopause (under the age of 40 years) (see Chapter 16).

A history of a recent endometrial curettage or endometritis in a patient with normal genitalia and normal endocrinology, but with absent or only a small withdrawal bleed following a progestogen challenge, is suggestive of Asherman syndrome. A hysteroscopy can confirm the diagnosis.

Measurement of bone mineral density (BMD) is indicated in amenorrhoeic women who are estrogen-deficient. Measurements of bone density are made in the lumbar spine and femoral neck. The vertebral

**Table 7.1    Classification of primary amenorrhoea**

| Organ/system | Cause |
|---|---|
| Uterus | Müllerian agenesis (e.g. Rokitansky syndrome) |
| Ovaries | Polycystic ovary syndrome<br>Premature ovarian failure (usually genetic, e.g. Turner syndrome)<br>Weight loss |
| Hypothalamus (hypogonadotrophic hypogonadism) | Intense exercise (e.g. ballerinas)<br>Idiopathic |
| Delayed puberty | Constitutional delay or secondary |
| Pituitary | Hyperprolactinaemia<br>Hypopituitarism |
| Hypothalamic/pituitary damage (hypogonadism) | Tumours (craniopharyngiomas, gliomas, germinomas, dermoid cysts)<br>Cranial irradiation, head injury (rare in young girls) |
| Systemic | Chronic debilitating illness<br>Weight loss<br>Endocrine disorders (thyroid disease, Cushing's syndrome, etc.) |

bone is more sensitive to estrogen deficiency and vertebral fractures tend to occur in a younger age group (50–60 years) than fractures at the femoral neck (70+ years). However, it should be noted that crush fractures can spuriously increase the measured BMD. An X-ray of the dorsolumbar spine is therefore often carried out, particularly in patients who have lost height.

Amenorrhoea may also have long-term metabolic and physical consequences. In women with PCOS and prolonged amenorrhoea, there is a risk of endometrial hyperplasia and adenocarcinoma. If, on resumption of menstruation, there is a history of persistent intermenstrual bleeding or if on ultrasound there is a postmenstrual endometrial thickness of greater than 10 mm, an endometrial biopsy is indicated (see Chapter 8).

Serum cholesterol measurements are important because of the association of an increased risk of heart disease in women with premature ovarian failure. Women with PCOS, although not estrogen-deficient, may have a subnormal HDL/total cholesterol ratio. This is a consequence of the hypersecretion of insulin that occurs in many women with PCOS and may increase the lifetime risk of heart disease (see Chapter 9).

# Causes of amenorrhoea

Many conditions that cause primary amenorrhoea will have presented either at birth or during childhood (Table 7.1). Management should be in a specialised clinic that can provide a multidisciplinary approach to care (see Chapter 1).

The principal causes of secondary amenorrhoea are outlined in Table 7.2. The frequency with which these conditions present is shown in Table 7.3.

## GENITAL TRACT ABNORMALITIES

Asherman syndrome is a condition in which intrauterine adhesions prevent normal growth of the endometrium. This may be the result of an excessively vigorous endometrial curettage, or it may follow endometritis. Typically, amenorrhoea is not absolute and it may be possible to induce a withdrawal bleed. Diagnosis and treatment by adhesiolysis is done hysteroscopically. Following surgery, a three-month course of cyclical

**Table 7.2    Classification of secondary amenorrhoea**

| Organ/system | Cause |
|---|---|
| Uterus | Asherman syndrome<br>Cervical stenosis |
| Ovaries | Polycystic ovary syndrome<br>Premature ovarian failure (genetic,<br>autoimmune, infective, radio/chemotherapy) |
| Hypothalamus (hypogonadotrophic hypogonadism) | Weight loss<br>Exercise<br>Chronic illness<br>Psychological distress<br>Idiopathic |
| Pituitary | Hyperprolactinaemia<br>Hypopituitarism<br>Sheehan syndrome |
| Hypothalamic/pituitary damage (hypogonadism) | Tumours (craniopharyngioma, glioma,<br>germinoma, dermoid cyst)<br>Cranial irradiation<br>Head injury<br>Sarcoidosis<br>Tuberculosis |
| Systemic | Chronic debilitating illness<br>Weight loss<br>Endocrine disorders (thyroid disease,<br>Cushing's syndrome, etc.) |

| Table 7.3 | The aetiology of secondary amenorrhoea in 570 women attending an endocrine clinic | |
| --- | --- |
| *Aetiology* | *Incidence (%)* |
| Polycystic ovary syndrome | 36.9 |
| Premature ovarian failure | 23.6 |
| Hyperprolactinaemia | 16.9 |
| Weight-related amenorrhoea | 9.8 |
| Hypogonadotrophic hypogonadism | 5.9 |
| Hypopituitarism | 4.4 |
| Exercise-related amenorrhoea | 2.5 |

combined progesterone and estrogen should be given. Some clinicians insert a Foley catheter into the uterine cavity for seven to ten days postoperatively or an intrauterine contraceptive device for two to three months, in order to prevent recurrence of adhesions.

Cervical stenosis is an occasional cause of secondary amenorrhoea. It was relatively common following a traditional cone biopsy for the treatment of cervical intraepithelial neoplasia. However, modern procedures such as laser and loop diathermy have fewer postoperative cervical complications. Treatment for cervical stenosis consists of careful cervical dilatation – the concurrent use of laparoscopy and ultrasound may help to prevent the inadvertent creation of a false passage.

## SYSTEMIC DISORDERS CAUSING SECONDARY AMENORRHOEA

Chronic disease may result in menstrual disorders as a consequence of the general disease state, weight loss or the effect of the disease process on the hypothalamic–pituitary axis. Furthermore, a chronic disease that leads to immobility, such as chronic obstructive airways disease, may increase the risk of amenorrhoea-associated osteoporosis.

In addition, certain diseases affect gonadal function directly. Women with chronic renal failure have a discordantly elevated LH, possibly as a consequence of impaired clearance. Prolactin is also elevated in these women, due to failure of the normal dopamine inhibition. Diabetes mellitus may result in functional hypothalamic–pituitary amenorrhoea and be associated with an increased risk of PCOS. Liver disease affects the level of circulating sex hormone-binding globulin (SHGB) and, thus, circulating free hormone levels, thereby disrupting the normal feedback mechanisms. Metabolism of various hormones, including testosterone, are also liver-dependent: both menstruation and fertility return after liver transplantation. Endocrine disorders such as thyrotoxicosis and Cushing's syndrome are commonly associated with gonadal dysfunction. Autoimmune endocrinopathies may be associated with premature ovarian failure, because of ovarian antibodies (see Chapter 16).

Management for these women should concentrate on the underlying systemic problem and on preventing complications of estrogen deficiency. If fertility is required, it is desirable to achieve maximal health and where possible to discontinue teratogenic drugs.

## WEIGHT-RELATED AMENORRHOEA

Weight can have profound effects on gonadotrophin regulation and release. Weight disorders are also common. In one study, up to 35% of women attending an endocrine clinic had secondary amenorrhoea associated with weight loss. A regular menstrual cycle is unlikely to occur if the BMI is less than 19 kg/m.$^2$ Fat appears to be critical to a normally functioning hypothalamic–pituitary–gonadal axis. It is estimated that at least 22% of body weight should be fat in order to maintain ovulatory cycles. This level enables the extra ovarian aromatisation of androgens to estrogens and maintains appropriate feedback control of the hypothalamic–pituitary–ovarian axis. Therefore, girls who are significantly underweight before puberty may have primary amenorrhoea, while those who are significantly underweight after puberty will have secondary amenorrhoea. To cause amenorrhoea, the loss must be 10–15% of the women's normal weight for height. Weight loss may be due to a number of causes, including self-induced abstinence, starvation, illness and exercise. However, whatever the precipitating cause, the net result is impairment of gonadotrophin secretion. Weight-related gonadotrophin deficiency results in a greater suppression of LH than FSH. Combined with the reduction in pulsatility of gonadotrophin secretion, this may result in a 'multicystic' pattern in the ovary. This appearance is typical of normal puberty and occurs when there are several cysts (about 5–10 mm in diameter together with a stroma of normal density).

Anorexia nervosa is at the extreme end of a spectrum of eating disorders and is invariably accompanied by menstrual disturbance and, indeed, may account for between 15% and 35% of women with amenorrhoea. Women with anorexia nervosa should be managed in collaboration with a psychiatrist, and it is essential to encourage weight gain as the main therapy.

An artificial cycle may be induced with the combined oral contraceptive. However, this may corroborate the denial of weight loss being the underlying problem. Similarly, although it is possible to induce ovulation with GnRH or exogenous gonadotrophins, treatment of infertility in the significantly underweight woman is associated with a significant increase in intrauterine growth restriction and neonatal problems. Low birthweight is also now being related to an increased risk of cardiovascular disease, obstructive lung disease and schizophrenia in adult life.

Weight-related amenorrhoea may also have profound long-term effects on bone mineral density. Estrogen deficiency, reduced calcium and protein intake, reduced levels of vitamin D and elevated cortisol levels can all contribute to osteoporosis. The age of onset of anorexia nervosa is also important, as prolonged amenorrhoea before the normal age at which peak bone mass is obtained (approximately 25 years) increases the likelihood of severe osteoporosis.

Worldwide, involuntary starvation is the most common cause of reduced reproductive ability, resulting in delayed pubertal growth and menarche in adolescents and infertility in adults. Acute malnutrition, as seen in famine conditions and during and after the Second World War, has profound effects on fertility and fecundity. Ovulatory function usually returns quickly on restoration of adequate nutrition. The chronic malnutrition common in developing countries has less profound effects on fertility but is associated with small and premature babies.

## LEPTIN

Leptin is a 167-amino-acid peptide that is secreted by fat cells in response to insulin and glucocorticoids. Leptin is transported by a protein that appears to be the extracellular domain of the leptin receptor itself. Leptin receptors are found in the choroid plexus, on the hypothalamus and ovary and at many other sites. Leptin decreases the intake of food and stimulates thermogenesis. Leptin also appears to inhibit the hypothalamic peptide neuropeptide-Y, which is an inhibitor of GnRH pulsatility. Leptin appears to serve a signal from the body fat to the brain about the adequacy of fat stores for reproduction. Thus, menstruation will occur only if fat stores are adequate. Obesity, on the other hand, is associated with high circulating concentrations of leptin and this in turn might be a mechanism for hypersecretion of LH in women with PCOS. To date, most studies have been in the leptin-deficient and consequently obese *Ob/Ob* mouse. Starvation of the *Ob/Ob* mouse leads to weight loss, yet fertility is only restored after the administration of leptin. Leptin administration to overweight infertile women may not be as straightforward as it might initially seem because of the complex nature of leptin transport into the brain (see Figure 3.4, Chapter 3).

## PSYCHOLOGICAL STRESS

Studies have failed to demonstrate a link between stressful life events and amenorrhoea of greater than two months. However, stress may lead to physical debility such as weight loss, which may then cause menstrual disturbance.

## EXERCISE-RELATED AMENORRHOEA

Menstrual disturbance is common in athletes undergoing intensive training. Between 10% and 20% have oligomenorrhoea or amenorrhoea, compared with 5% in the general population. Amenorrhoea is more common in athletes aged under 30 years of age and is particularly common in women involved in endurance events (such as long-distance running). Up to 50% of competitive runners training 80 miles per week may be amenorrhoeic.

The main aetiological factors are weight and percentage body fat content, but other factors have also been postulated. Physiological changes are consistent with those associated with starvation and chronic illness. In order to conserve energy, there may be a fall in thyroid-stimulating hormone (TSH), a reduction in triiodothyronine ($T_3$) and an elevation of the inactive reverse-$T_3$. Exercise also leads to a fall in circulating insulin and IGF-1 and therefore decreases their stimulation of the pituitary and ovary.

Ballet dancers provide an interesting and much studied subgroup of sportswomen because their training begins at an early age. They have been found to have a significant delay in menarche (15.4 years compared with 12.5 years) and a restriction in pubertal development that parallels the intensity of their training. Menstrual irregularities are common and up to 44% have secondary amenorrhoea. In a survey of 75 dancers, 61% were found to have stress fractures and 24% had scoliosis. The risk of these pathological features was increased if menarche was delayed or if there were prolonged periods of amenorrhoea. These findings may be explained by delayed pubertal maturation resulting in attainment of a greater than expected height and a predisposition to scoliosis, as estrogen is required for epiphyseal closure.

Exercise-induced amenorrhoea has the potential to cause severe long-term morbidity, particularly with regard to osteoporosis. Studies on young ballet dancers have shown that the amount of exercise undertaken by these dancers does not compensate for these osteoporotic changes. Estrogen is also important in the formation of collagen and soft tissue injuries are also common in dancers.

Whereas moderate exercise has been found to reduce the incidence of postmenopausal osteoporosis, young athletes may be placing themselves at risk at an age when the attainment of peak bone mass is important for long-term skeletal strength. Appropriate advice should be given, particularly regarding diet, and the use of a cyclical estrogen/progestogen preparation should be considered. It is important to enlist the support of both parents and trainers when trying to encourage a young athlete to modify her exercise programme and diet in order to reinstate a normal menstrual cycle with the aim of preventing long-term morbidity.

## HYPOTHALAMIC CAUSES OF SECONDARY AMENORRHOEA

Hypothalamic causes of amenorrhoea may be either primary or secondary. Primary hypothalamic lesions include craniopharyngiomas, germinomas, gliomas and dermoid cysts. These hypothalamic lesions either disrupt the normal pathway of prolactin inhibitory factor (dopamine), thus causing hyperprolactinaemia or compress and/or destroy hypothalamic and pituitary tissue. Treatment is usually surgical, with additional radiotherapy if required. Hormone replacement therapy is required to mimic ovarian function and, if the pituitary gland is damaged either by the lesion or by the treatment, replacement thyroid and adrenal hormones are required.

Secondary hypogonadotrophic hypogonadism may result from systemic conditions, including sarcoidosis and tuberculosis, as well as head injury or cranial irradiation. Sheehan syndrome, the result of profound and prolonged hypotension on the sensitive pituitary gland, enlarged by pregnancy, may also be a cause of hypogonadotrophic hypogonadism in a woman with a history of a major obstetric haemorrhage. It is essential to assess the pituitary function fully in all these women and then instigate the appropriate replacement therapy. Ovulation may be induced with pulsatile subcutaneous GnRH or hMG. The administration of pulsatile GnRH provides the most 'physiological' correction of infertility caused by hypogonadotrophic hypogonadism and results in unifollicular ovulation (provided, of course, that the pituitary gland is intact), while hMG therapy requires close monitoring to prevent multiple pregnancy. Purified or recombinant FSH preparations are not suitable for women with hypogonadotrophic hypogonadism (or pituitary hypogonadism), as these patients have absent endogenous production of LH and so although follicular growth may occur, estrogen biosynthesis is impaired. Thus, hMG, which contains FSH and LH activity, is necessary for these patients.

## PITUITARY CAUSES OF SECONDARY AMENORRHOEA

Hyperprolactinaemia is the most common pituitary cause of amenorrhoea (see Chapter 12). This may be physiological, as during lactation, iatrogenic or pathological. A nonfunctioning tumour in the region of the hypothalamus or pituitary, which disrupts the inhibitory influence of dopamine on prolactin secretion, and pituitary adenomas will both cause hyperprolactinomas. Other known causes are certain drugs, particularly prothiazines and metoclopramide, which act as dopamine antagonists.

In women with amenorrhoea associated with hyperprolactinaemia, the main symptoms are usually those of estrogen deficiency. Galactorrhoea may be found in up to one-third of women with hypoprolactinaemia, although its appearance is correlated neither with prolactin levels nor with the presence of a tumour. Approximately 5% of women present with visual field defects. For ovarian causes of amenorrhoea see Chapter 8 (polycystic ovary syndrome) and Chapter 16 (premature ovarian failure).

## IATROGENIC CAUSES OF AMENORRHOEA

There are many iatrogenic causes of amenorrhoea, which may be either temporary or permanent. These include malignant conditions that require either radiation to the abdomen or pelvis or chemotherapy. Both of these treatments may result in permanent gonadal damage. The amount of damage is related directly to the woman's age, the cumulative dose and the woman's prior menstrual status.

Gynaecological procedures involving oophorectomy will inevitably result in estrogen deficiency and amenorrhoea. Hormone replacement should be prescribed for these women where appropriate.

---

**SECONDARY AMENORRHOEA KEY POINTS**

- Secondary amenorrhoea is usually considered to be amenorrhoea of six or more months' duration during reproductive years.
- Aetiology and treatment can be conveniently categorised into hypothalamic, pituitary, ovarian, uterine causes or systemic illness, which in essence causes secondary hypothalamic amenorrhoea.
- Correct diagnosis is readily made if a logical protocol is applied.
- PCOS is the most common cause and is the only major cause of amenorrhoea that is not associated with estrogen deficiency.
- The amenorrhoea of PCOS should be treated in order to either enhance fertility or prevent endometrial hyperplasia and adenocarcinoma.
- Estrogen deficiency results in the long-term sequelae of osteoporosis and cardiovascular disease and so the cause of amenorrhoea should be corrected early and hormone replacement therapy administered if necessary.
- Fertility can be achieved either after ovulation induction or, in cases of premature ovarian failure, with oocyte donation/*in vitro* fertilisation.

---

Hormone therapy itself can be used to disrupt the menstrual cycle. However, iatrogenic causes of ovarian quiescence have the same consequences of estrogen deficiency due to any other aetiology. Thus, the use of GnRH analogues in the treatment of estrogen-dependent conditions (e.g. precocious puberty, endometriosis, uterine fibroids) results in a significant decrease in bone mineral density in as little as six months. However, the demineralisation is reversible with the cessation of therapy, especially for the treatment of benign conditions in young women who are in the process of achieving their peak bone mass. The concurrent use of an androgenic progestogen may protect against bone loss.

# 8  Polycystic ovary syndrome

Polycystic ovary syndrome (PCOS) is the most common endocrine disturbance that affects women; yet it is only in recent times that we have begun to piece together a clearer idea of its pathogenesis. PCOS is a heterogeneous collection of signs and symptoms that, gathered together, form a spectrum of a disorder with a mild presentation in some, while in others it presents as a severe disturbance of reproductive, endocrine and metabolic function. The pathophysiology of PCOS appears to be multifactorial and polygenic. The definition of the syndrome has been much debated. Key features include menstrual cycle disturbance, hyperandrogenism and obesity. There are many extra-ovarian aspects to the pathophysiology of PCOS but ovarian dysfunction is central. At a joint consensus meeting of the European Society of Human Reproduction and Embryology (ESHRE) and the American Society for Reproductive Medicine (ASRM), a refined definition of the PCOS was agreed: the presence of two out of the following three criteria:

- oligo- and/or anovulation
- hyperandrogenism (clinical and/or biochemical)
- polycystic ovaries, with the exclusion of other aetiologies.[1]

The morphology of the polycystic ovary has been redefined as an ovary with 12 or more follicles measuring 2–9 mm in diameter and/or increased ovarian volume (greater than 10 cm$^3$).[2]

There is considerable heterogeneity of symptoms and signs in women with PCOS (Box 8.1) and for an individual these may change over time.[3] Polycystic ovaries can exist without clinical signs of the syndrome, expression of which may be precipitated by various factors, predominantly an increase in body weight.

Genetic studies have identified a link between PCOS and disordered insulin metabolism, and indicate that the syndrome may be the presentation of a complex genetic trait disorder.[4] The features of obesity, hyperinsulinaemia and hyperandrogenaemia, which are commonly seen in PCOS, are also known to be factors that confer an increased risk of cardiovascular disease and type 2 diabetes mellitus.[5] There are studies that indicate that women with PCOS have an increased risk for these diseases that pose long-

## BOX 8.1 THE SPECTRUM OF CLINICAL MANIFESTATIONS OF THE POLYCYSTIC OVARY SYNDROME

### SYMPTOMS

- Hyperandrogenism (acne, hirsutism, alopecia)
- Menstrual disturbance (oligomenorrhoea, amenorrhoea)
- Infertility (even if cycles are regular and ovulatory)
- Obesity is not caused by having PCOS but will exacerbate its symptoms
- Asymptomatic, with polycystic ovaries on ultrasound scan

### ENDOCRINE AND METABOLIC DISTURBANCE

- ↑ Androgens (testosterone and androstenone)
- ↑ Luteinising hormone, normal or slightly reduced follicle-stimulating hormone
- ↑ Estradiol, estone (not routinely measured)
- ↓ Sex hormone-binding globulin, results in elevated 'free androgen index'; a good surrogate marker for hyperisnulinaemia
- ↑ Fasting insulin (not routinely measured; insulin resistance assessed by fasting glucose, sometimes combined with insulin or an oral 75-g glucose tolerance test (GTT) to assess impaired glucose tolerance)
- ↑ Prolactin

### POSSIBLE LATE SEQUELAE

- Diabetes mellitus
- Dyslipidaemia
- Hypertension
- Cardiovascular disease
- Endometrial carcinoma
- Breast cancer

term risks for health and this evidence has prompted debate as to the need for screening women for polycystic ovaries. Because the phenotype of women with polycystic ovaries and the polycystic ovary syndrome may be very variable[3] it is then difficult to elucidate the genotype. It is also likely that different combinations of genetic variants may result in differential expression of the separate components of the syndrome.[6]

The highest reported prevalence of polycystic ovaries has been 52% among South Asian immigrants in Britain, of whom 49.1% had menstrual irregularity.[7] This study demonstrated that South Asian women with polycystic ovaries had a comparable degree of insulin resistance to controls with established type 2 diabetes mellitus. Generally, there has been a paucity of data of the prevalence of PCOS among women of South Asian origin, both among migrant and native groups. Type 2 diabetes and insulin resistance have a high prevalence among indigenous populations in South Asia, with a rising prevalence among women. Insulin resistance and hyperinsulinaemia are common antecedents of type 2 diabetes, with a high prevalence in South Asians. Type 2 diabetes also has a familial basis, inherited as a complex genetic trait that interacts with environmental factors, chiefly nutrition, commencing from fetal life. We have already found that South Asian women with anovular PCOS have greater insulin resistance and more severe symptoms of the syndrome than anovular white women with PCOS.[8] Furthermore, it has been found that women from South Asia living in the UK appear to express symptoms at an earlier age than their white British counterparts.[8]

## Pathogenesis

High-resolution ultrasound scanning has made possible an accurate estimate of the prevalence of polycystic ovaries. Several studies have estimated the prevalence of polycystic ovaries in 'normal adult' women and found rates of 22–33% but it is not known at what age they first appear.[9,10] PCOS appears to have its origins during adolescence and is thought to be associated with increased weight gain during puberty. However, the polycystic ovary gene(s) has not been identified and the effects of environmental influences, such as weight change, circulating hormone concentrations and the age at which these occur, are still being unravelled.

Many women with polycystic ovaries detected by ultrasound do not have overt symptoms of PCOS, although symptoms may develop later, after a gain in weight, for example. Ovarian morphology using the ultrasound criteria described by Adams et al.[11] (ten or more cysts, 2–8 mm in diameter, arranged around an echo dense stroma, as seen by transabdominal scan; Figures 8.1, 8.2, 8.3) appears to be the most sensitive diagnostic marker for polycystic ovaries. The polycystic ovary has been redefined by transvaginal ultrasound as an ovary with 12 or more follicles measuring 2–9 mm in diameter and/or increased ovarian volume (greater than 10 cm$^3$).[3] It is known that obesity is not a prerequisite for PCOS. Indeed, in a series of 1741 women with polycystic ovaries in a study by Balen et al.,[3] only 38.4% of women were overweight (BMI greater than 25 kg/m$^2$). The multicystic ovary (Figure 8.4) has normal stroma and is seen typically during puberty and the recovery phase of hypothalamic amenorrhoea.

### GENETICS OF POLYCYSTIC OVARY SYNDROME

PCOS runs in families, with approximately 50% of first-degree female relatives (sisters and mothers) also having PCOS. A number of candidate

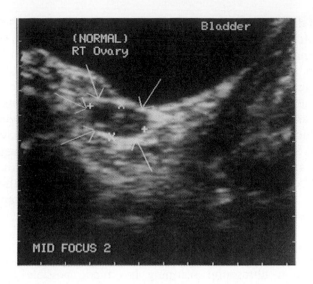

**Figure 8.1** Transabdominal ultrasound scan of a normal ovary; reproduced with permission of Churchill Livingstone from Balen and Jacobs, *Infertility in Practice*, 2003

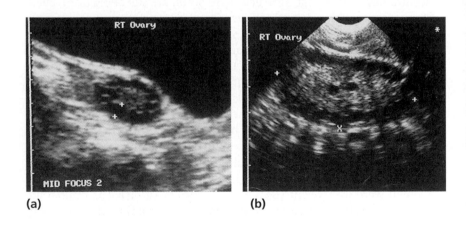

(a)                                            (b)

**Figure 8.2** **(a)** Transabdominal and **(b)** transvaginal ultrasound scans of a polycystic ovary; reproduced with permission of Churchill Livingstone from Balen and Jacobs, *Infertility in Practice*, 2003

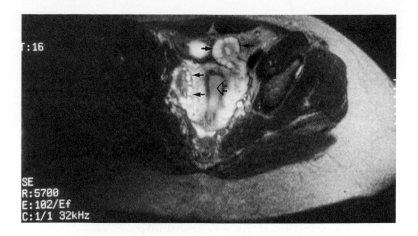

**Figure 8.3** Magnetic resonance imaging of a pelvis, demonstrating two polycystic ovaries (closed arrows) and a hyperplastic endometrium (open arrow); reproduced with permission of Churchill Livingstone from Balen and Jacobs, *Infertility in Practice*, 2003

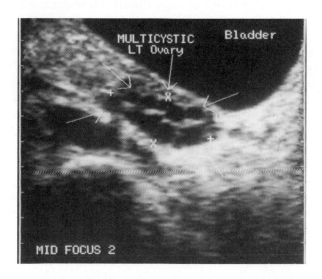

**Figure 8.4** Transabdominal ultrasound scan of a multicystic ovary; reproduced with permission of Churchill Livingstone from Balen and Jacobs, *Infertility in Practice*, 2003

**Table 8.1** Clinical signs and symptoms in women with polycystic ovary syndrome; n = 1741 (reproduced with permission from *Human Reproduction*[4])

| Sign or symptom | Occurrence (%) |
| --- | --- |
| Menstrual cycle disturbance: | |
|     Oligomenorrhoea | 47 |
|     Amenorrhoea | 19 |
| Hirsutism | 66 |
| Obesity | 38 |
| Acne | 34 |
| Infertility | 20 |
| Alopecia | 6 |
| Acanthosis nigricans | 2 |

genes have been proposed and research is continuing to unravel the genetics of PCOS. Earlier studies concentrated on disturbances of the control of androgen and gonadotropin secretion, while more recent work has focused on links with insulin secretion and insulin action.[12,13]

## HETEROGENEITY OF POLYCYSTIC OVARY SYNDROME

The findings of a large series of more than 1700 women with polycystic ovaries detected by ultrasound scan are summarised in Table 8.1.[3] All patients had at least one symptom of PCOS. Thirty-eight percent of the women were overweight (BMI greater than 25 kg/m²). Obesity was significantly associated with an increased risk of hirsutism, menstrual cycle disturbance and an elevated serum testosterone concentration. Obesity was also associated with an increased rate of infertility and menstrual cycle disturbance. Twenty-six percent of women with primary infertility and 14% of women with secondary infertility had a BMI of more than 30 kg/m.²

Approximately 30% of the women had a regular menstrual cycle, 50% had oligomenorrhoea and 20% had amenorrhoea. A rising serum concentration of testosterone was associated with an increased risk of hirsutism, infertility and cycle disturbance. The rates of infertility and menstrual cycle disturbance also increased with increasing serum LH concentrations greater than 10 iu/l. The serum LH concentration of those with primary infertility was significantly higher than that of women with secondary infertility and both were higher than the LH concentration of those with proven fertility. Ovarian morphology appears to be the most sensitive marker of PCOS, compared with the classical endocrine features of raised serum LH and testosterone, which were found in only 39.8% and 28.9% of women, respectively, in this series.

The key features of PCOS are ovarian hyperandrogenism and a disruption of normal folliculogenesis, which results in the multiple immature follicles within the ovaries. Androgen production by the theca cells is stimulated both by LH and insulin. Women with PCOS who are slim tend to have LH as the main driver of androgen excess while in women who are obese hyperinsulinaemia augments the effect of LH on the ovary. An elevated serum LH concentration has been associated with reduced reproductive outcome (reduced fertility and increased risk of miscarriage) even in women who are ovulating. Women with menstrual irregularity are more likely to have hyperinsulinaemia and it has been shown that the greater the interval between the periods of a woman with PCOS the greater her degree of insulin resistance.

# Management of polycystic ovary syndrome

## OBESITY

The clinical management of a woman with PCOS should be focused on her individual problems. Obesity worsens both symptomatology and the endocrine profile and obese women should therefore be encouraged to

| Table 8.2 | Investigations for polycystic ovary syndrome | |
|---|---|---|
| Test | Normal range[a] | Purpose/additional points |
| Pelvic ultrasound | | To test ovarian morphology and endometrial thickness; transabdominal scan satisfactory in women who are not sexually active |
| Testosterone (T) <br> Sex hormone-binding globulin (SHBG) | 0.5–3.5 nmol/l <br> 16–119 nmol/l | Unnecessary to measure other androgens unless total T > 5 nmol/l, in which case referral is indicated |
| Free androgen index (FAI): T x 100/SHGB | < 5 | Insulin suppresses SHBG, resulting in a high FAI in the presence of a normal total T |
| Estradiol | | Measurement is unhelpful to diagnosis |
| Luteinising hormone (LH) <br> Follicle-stimulating hormone (FSH) | 2–10 iu/l <br> 2–8 iu/l | FSH and LH are best measured during days 1–3 of a menstrual bleed. If oligo- or amenorrhoeic, then random samples are taken |
| Prolactin, thyroid function, thyroid-stimulating hormone | < 30 mu/l | Measure if oligo- or amenorrhoeic |

[a] May vary with local laboratory assays

lose weight. It has been suggested that rather than BMI itself, it is the distribution of fat that is important, with android obesity being more of a risk factor than gynecoid obesity; hence, the value of measuring waist-to-hip ratio or waist circumference, which detects abdominal visceral fat rather than subcutaneous fat (the waist circumference of a woman should be less than 88 cm). It is the visceral fat that is metabolically active and, when increased, results in increased rates of insulin resistance, type 2 diabetes, dyslipidaemia, hypertension and left ventricular enlargement. Exercise has a significant effect on reducing visceral fat and reducing cardiovascular risk; a 5% reduction in body weight may lead to a 30% reduction in visceral fat.

Elevated serum concentrations of insulin are more common in both lean and obese women with PCOS than weight-matched controls. Indeed it is hyperinsulinaemia that appears to be the key to the pathogenesis of the syndrome, as insulin stimulates androgen secretion by the ovarian stroma and appears to affect the normal development of ovarian follicles, both by the adverse effects of androgens on follicular growth and possibly also by suppressing apoptosis and permitting the survival of follicles otherwise destined to disappear. The prevalence of diabetes in women with PCOS who are obese is at least 11% and so a measurement of impaired glucose tolerance is important and long-term screening advisable.

Insulin resistance is defined as a diminution in the biological responses to a given level of insulin. In the presence of an adequate pancreatic reserve, normal circulating glucose levels are maintained at higher serum insulin concentrations. There have been a large number of studies demonstrating the presence of insulin resistance and corresponding hyperinsulinaemia in both obese and non-obese women with PCOS. Women with PCOS who are obese have consistently been shown to be insulin-resistant to a greater degree than their weight-matched controls. It appears that obesity and PCOS have a synergistic effect on the degree and severity of the insulin resistance and subsequent hyperinsulinaemia

**Table 8.3** Definitions of glucose tolerance after a 75-g glucose tolerance test (GTT)

|  | Diabetes mellitus | Impaired glucose tolerance | Impaired fasting glycaemia |
|---|---|---|---|
| Fasting glucose (mmol/l) | ≥ 7.0 | < 7.0 | ≥ 6.1 and < 7.0 |
| 2-hour glucose | ≤ 11.1 | ≥ 7.8 – ≤ 11.1 | < 7.8 |
| Action | Refer to diabetic clinic | Dietary advice; check fasting glucose annually | Dietary advice; check fasting glucose annually |

in this group of women. Insulin resistance correlates both with intermenstrual interval and with hyperandrogenaemia.

Women who are obese, and also many slim women with PCOS, will have insulin resistance and elevated serum concentrations of insulin (usually less than 30 mu/l fasting). It is suggested that a 75-g oral GTT be performed in women with PCOS and a BMI greater than 30 kg/m², with an assessment of the fasting and two-hour glucose concentration. It has been suggested that South Asian women should have an assessment of glucose tolerance if their BMI is greater than 25 kg/m² because of the greater risk of insulin resistance at a lower BMI than seen in the white population (Table 8.3).

Exercise and weight loss have so far been the most physiological way to improve insulin sensitivity and improve the metabolic abnormalities associated with the syndrome. In women with PCOS it has been demonstrated that even partial weight loss improves the hormonal profile and improvement in the reproductive outcome for all forms of fertility treatment. Since the association between insulin resistance and BMI is stronger in obese women with PCOS than in weight-matched controls, the benefits of weight loss should be even greater in these women than in women without PCOS. Women should therefore be advised on appropriate diet combined with adequate exercise. There is no evidence that one particular type of diet is preferable, although inherently those with a low glycaemic index may be beneficial.

Anti-obesity drugs may help with weight loss and both orlistat and sibutramine have been shown to be effective in PCOS in small studies. Both agents can also improve insulin sensitivity and are currently licensed for individuals with a BMI greater than 30 kg/m² or lower if comorbidities such as hyperlipidaemia are present. Both agents have been shown to improve insulin resistance and orlistat has been shown to reduce testosterone. These drugs can be prescribed by general practitioners but their use must be monitored, particularly the woman's blood pressure with sibutramine.

Insulin-sensitising agents such as metformin have become increasingly popular in the management of PCOS (see also Chapter 9) as it was thought that they acted directly at the pathogenesis of the syndrome and helped to correct both metabolic and endocrine problems. Early studies suggested an improvement in reproductive function and menstrual cycle regulation, although large prospective studies have not confirmed a major benefit and certainly not with respect to achieving weight loss.

## MENSTRUAL IRREGULARITY

In women with anovulatory cycles, the action of estradiol on the endometrium is unopposed because of the lack of cyclical progesterone secretion. This may result in episodes of irregular uterine bleeding and, in the long term, endometrial hyperplasia and even endometrial cancer. The easiest way to control the menstrual cycle is by use of a low-dose combined oral contraceptive preparation. This will result in an artificial cycle and regular shedding of the endometrium. It is also important once again to encourage weight loss. As women with PCOS are thought to be at increased risk of cardiovascular disease, a 'lipid-friendly' combined contraceptive pill should be used. An alternative is a progestogen (such as medroxyprogesterone acetate or dydrogesterone) taken for 12 days every one to three months to induce a withdrawal bleed.

An ultrasound assessment of endometrial thickness provides a bioassay for estradiol production by the ovaries and conversion of androgens in the peripheral fat. If the endometrium is thicker than 15 mm, a withdrawal bleed should be induced and, if the endometrium fails to shed, endometrial sampling is required to exclude endometrial hyperplasia or malignancy. The only young women to develop endometrial carcinoma (age less than 35 years), which otherwise has a mean age of occurrence of 61 years in the UK, are those with anovulation secondary to PCOS or estrogen-secreting tumours.

## INFERTILITY

See Chapter 10 for the management of infertility in PCOS.

## HYPERANDROGENISM AND HIRSUTISM

The bioavailability of testosterone is affected by the serum concentration of SHBG. High levels of insulin lower the production of SHBG and so increase the free fraction of androgen. Elevated serum androgen concentrations stimulate peripheral androgen receptors, resulting in an increase in 5α-reductase activity, directly increasing the conversion of testosterone to the more potent metabolite dihydrotestosterone. Symptoms of hyperandrogenism include hirsutism, which can be a distressing condition. Hirsutism is characterised by terminal hair growth in a male pattern of distribution, including chin, upper lip, chest, upper and lower back, upper and lower abdomen, upper arm, thigh and buttocks. A standardised scoring system, such as the modified Ferriman and Gallwey score, should be used to evaluate the degree of hirsutism before and during treatments (Figure 8.5).

Treatment options include cosmetic and medical therapies. Medical regimens halt the progression of hirsutism and decrease the rate of hair growth. However, drug therapies may take six to nine months or longer before any benefit is perceived and so physical treatments, including electrolysis, laser treatment, waxing and bleaching, may be helpful while

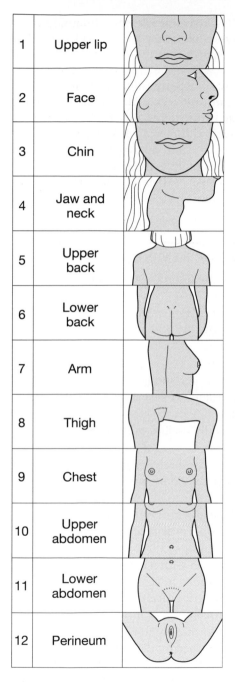

| 1 | Upper lip |
| 2 | Face |
| 3 | Chin |
| 4 | Jaw and neck |
| 5 | Upper back |
| 6 | Lower back |
| 7 | Arm |
| 8 | Thigh |
| 9 | Chest |
| 10 | Upper abdomen |
| 11 | Lower abdomen |
| 12 | Perineum |

**Figure 8.5** Ferriman Gallwey score

waiting for medical treatments to work. Topical eflornithine is proving also to be efficacious. It works by inhibiting the enzyme ornithine decarboxylase in hair follicles and may be a useful therapy for those who wish to avoid hormonal treatments. The management of alopecia is much harder and may require a combination of oral anti-androgens and topical minoxidil.

Symptoms of hyperandrogenism can be treated by a combination of an estrogen (such as ethinylestradiol or a combined contraceptive pill) and the antiandrogen cyproterone acetate (50–100 mg). Estrogens lower circulating androgens by a combination of a slight inhibition of gonadotrophin secretion and gonadotrophin-sensitive ovarian steroid production and by an increase in hepatic production of SHBG, resulting in lower free testosterone. The cyproterone is taken for the first ten days of a cycle (the 'reversed sequential' method) and the estrogen for the first 21 days. After a gap of exactly seven days, during which menstruation usually occurs, the regimen is repeated. As an alternative, the preparation cocyprindiol contains ethinylestradiol in combination with cyproterone, although at a lower dose (2 mg). Cyproterone acetate acts as a competitive inhibitor at the androgen receptor. Cyproterone acetate can occasionally cause liver damage and liver function should be checked regularly. Other anti-androgens such as ketoconazole and flutamide have been tried but because of their adverse effects they are not widely used in the UK. Spironolactone, a potassium-sparing diuretic, has anti-androgenic properties and is useful in women for whom the oral contraceptive pill is contraindicated (for example, because of hypertension). One preparation, Yasmin® (Schering Health Care Ltd, Burgess Hill, Sussex), contains ethinylestradiol and a progestogen, drospirenone (a derivative of spironolactone). This combined oral contraceptive is showing early promise for the management of PCOS. The anti-androgen finasteride may be useful for resistant cases. Other anti-androgens such as ketoconazole and flutamide have been tried but because of their adverse effects are not recommended for use in the UK. Metformin may also benefit some

---

**POLYCYSTIC OVARY SYNDROME KEY POINTS**

- PCOS is the most common endocrine disorder in women (approximate prevalence 10–15%).
- PCOS is a heterogeneous condition. Diagnosis is made by the ultrasound detection of polycystic ovaries and one or more of a combination of symptoms and signs.
- Management is symptom-orientated.
- If obese, weight loss improves symptoms and endocrinology and should be encouraged. A glucose tolerance test should be performed if the BMI is greater than 30 kg/m$^2$.
- Menstrual cycle control is achieved by cyclical oral contraceptives or progestogens.
- Ovulation induction may be difficult and require progression through various treatments, which should be monitored carefully to prevent multiple pregnancy.
- Ovulation induction may be achieved with clomiphene citrate, gonadotrophin therapy or laparoscopic ovarian diathermy (see Chapter 10).
- Hyperandrogenism is usually managed with a combined oral contraceptive containing ethinylestradiol in combination with cyproterone acetate (Dianette®, Schering Health). Alternatives include Yasmin® (Schering Health), spironolactone and finasteride.
- Insulin-sensitising agents (e.g. metformin) require further long-term evaluation and should only be prescribed by endocrinologists and reproductive endocrinologists.

women with hyperandrogenism but this drug has not been proven to be the panacea that was originally hoped.

# References

1. The Rotterdam ESHRE/ASRM-sponsored PCOS consensus workshop group. Revised 2003 consensus on diagnostic criteria and long-term health risks related to polycystic ovary syndrome (PCOS). *Hum Reprod* 2004;**19**:41–7.

2. Balen AH, Laven JSE, Tan SL, Dewailly D. Ultrasound assessment of the polycystic ovary: international consensus definitions. *Hum Reprod Update* 2003;**9**:505–14.

3 Balen AH, Conway GS, Kaltsas G, Techatraisak K, Manning PJ, West C, Jacobs HS. Polycystic ovary syndrome: the spectrum of the disorder in 1741 patients. *Hum Reprod* 1995;**10**:2107–11.

4 Franks S, Gharani N, McCarthy M. Candidate genes in polycystic ovary syndrome. *Human Reprod Update* 2001;**7**:405–10.

5 Rajkowha M, Glass MR, Rutherford AJ, Michelmore K, Balen AH. Polycystic ovary syndrome: a risk factor for cardiovascular disease? *BJOG* 2000;**107**:11–18.

6 Balen AH, Michelmore K. What is polycystic ovary syndrome? Are national views important? *Hum Reprod* 2002;**17**:2219–27.

7 Rodin DA, Bano G, Bland JM, Taylor K, Nussey SS. Polycystic ovaries and associated metabolic abnormalities in Indian subcontinent Asian women. *Clin Endocrinol* 1998;**49**:91–9.

8 Wijeyaratne CN, Balen AH, Barth J, Belchetz PE. Clinical manifestations and insulin resistance (IR) in polycystic ovary syndrome (PCOS) among South Asians and Caucasians: is there a difference? *Clin Endocrinol* 2002;**57**:343–50.

9 Polson DW, Adams J, Wadsworth J, Franks S. Polycystic ovaries: a common finding in normal women. *Lancet* 1988;**1**:870–72.

10 Michelmore KF, Balen AH, Dunger DB, Vessey MP. Polycystic ovaries and associated clinical and biochemical features in young women. *Clin Endocrinol (Oxf)* 1999;**51**:779–86.

11 Adams J, Franks S, Polson DW, Mason HD, Abdulwahid N, Tucker M, *et al.* Multifollicular ovaries: clinical and endocrine features and response to pulsatile gonadotrophin releasing hormone. *Lancet* 1985;**2**:1375–9.

12 Balen AH. The pathogenesis of polycystic ovary syndrome: the enigma unravels? *Lancet* 1999;**354**:966–7.

13 Waterworth DM, Bennett ST, Gharani N, McCarthy MI, Hague S, Batty S, *et al.* Linkage and association of insulin gene VNTR regulatory polymorphism with polycystic ovary syndrome. *Lancet* 1997;**349**:986–90.

# 9 Health consequences of polycystic ovary syndrome

The long-term risks of endometrial hyperplasia and endometrial carcinoma due to chronic anovulation and unopposed estrogen have long been recognised. With increasing awareness of the metabolic abnormalities associated with the syndrome, there is concern regarding cardiovascular risk and other long-term health implications in these women.

Obesity and metabolic abnormalities are recognised risk factors for the development of ischaemic heart disease (IHD) in the general population and these are also recognised features of PCOS. IHD accounts for 18% of deaths in men and 14% of deaths in women in Europe. In men, the incidence of IHD increases after the age of 35 years, while in women an increased incidence is noted after the age of 55 years.

Women with PCOS may be at greater risk for cardiovascular disease because they are more insulin-resistant than weight-matched controls and the metabolic disturbances associated with insulin resistance are known to increase cardiovascular risk in other populations.

## Insulin resistance

Insulin resistance is defined as a diminution in the biological responses to a given level of insulin. In the presence of an adequate pancreatic reserve, normal circulating glucose levels are maintained at higher serum insulin concentrations.

In the general population, cardiovascular risk factors include insulin resistance, obesity, glucose intolerance, hypertension and dyslipidaemia. A prospective population-based study of 1462 women aged between 38 and 60 years was undertaken in Gothenberg, Sweden, to examine cardiovascular risk factors in women.[1] After a 12-year follow-up, they reported four independent risk factors for myocardial infarction in women, which included increased waist-to-hip ratio, raised serum triglyceride concentrations, diabetes and hypertension. A further follow-up of the same cohort of women for a period of 20 years found that the two most important factors relating to cardiovascular mortality were central obesity and raised serum triglycerides. Central obesity was a more important risk factor than obesity itself.

Two large American epidemiological studies on heart disease in women – the Framingham and Lipid Research Clinic Follow-up studies – demonstrated that the mortality from cardiovascular disease was closely related to the lipid fractions, namely elevated serum triglycerides and reduced high-density lipoprotein (HDL) cholesterol levels. In 1988, Reaven[2] described 'syndrome X', or the insulin resistance syndrome, which is characterised by the presence of hyperinsulinaemia, varying degrees of glucose intolerance, dyslipidaemia, central obesity and hypertension. It was suggested that the metabolic and haemodynamic abnormalities associated with syndrome X constitute a major role in the aetiology and risk factors leading to coronary heart disease.

## Insulin resistance in polycystic ovary syndrome

Burghen et al.[3] made the first suggestion of a relationship between the hyperandrogenism of PCOS and hyperinsulinaemia. There was a significant correlation between basal insulin measurements with both serum testosterone and androstenedione concentrations. Subsequently, the presence of hyperinsulinaemia has been demonstrated in women with PCOS who are not obese, in order to demonstrate that this was a feature specific to PCOS rather than secondary to obesity. Since then, there have been a large number of studies demonstrating the presence of insulin resistance and corresponding hyperinsulinaemia in both obese and non-obese women with PCOS. Obese women with PCOS have consistently been shown to be insulin-resistant to a greater degree than their weight-matched controls. It appears that obesity and PCOS appear to have a synergistic effect on the degree and severity of the insulin resistance and subsequent hyperinsulinaemia in this group of women.

Insulin sensitivity varies depending upon menstrual pattern. Women with PCOS who are oligomenorrhoeic are more likely to be insulin-resistant than those with regular cycles, irrespective of their BMI.

## Other risk factors for ischaemic heart disease in women with polycystic ovary syndrome

### CENTRAL OBESITY

Simple obesity is associated with greater deposition of gluteofemoral fat while central obesity involves greater truncal abdominal fat distribution. Obesity is observed in 35–60% of women with PCOS. Hyperandrogenism is associated with a preponderance of fat localised to truncal abdominal sites. Women with PCOS have a greater truncal abdominal fat distribution as demonstrated by a higher waist-to-hip ratio. The central distribution of fat is independent of BMI and associated with higher plasma insulin and triglyceride concentrations and reduced HDL cholesterol concentrations.

## IMPAIRED GLUCOSE TOLERANCE AND DIABETES

These are known risk factors for cardiovascular disease. It is reported that 18–20% of obese women with PCOS demonstrate impaired glucose tolerance. Dahlgren *et al.*[4] noted the prevalence of type 2 diabetes was 15% in women with PCOS compared with 2% in controls. Insulin resistance combined with abdominal obesity is thought to account for the higher prevalence of type 2 diabetes in PCOS. There is a concomitant increased risk of gestational diabetes.

## HYPERTENSION

The prevalence of treated hypertension is three times higher in women with PCOS between the ages of 40 and 59 years compared with controls.[3] Gjonnaess[5] reported the incidence of pre-eclampsia in obese women with PCOS conceiving after ovarian electrocautery to be 12.9% compared with 3.8% in the general pregnant population.

## DYSLIPIDAEMIA

Women with PCOS have high concentrations of serum triglycerides and suppressed HDL levels, particularly a lower $HDL_2$ subfraction. HDLs play an important role in lipid metabolism and are the most important lipid parameter in predicting cardiovascular risk in women (see Chapter 15). HDLs perform the task of 'reverse cholesterol transport'. That is, they remove excess lipids from the circulation and tissues to transport them to the liver for excretion, or transfer them to other lipoprotein particles. Cholesterol is only one component of HDL, a particle with constantly changing composition forming $HDL_3$ and then $HDL_2$, as unesterified cholesterol is taken from tissue, esterified and exchanged for triglyceride with other lipoprotein species. Consequently, measurement of a single constituent in a particle involved in a dynamic process gives an incomplete picture.

In a detailed study of HDL composition it was found that obesity was the most important factor associated with elevated serum total triglyceride, cholesterol and phospholipid concentrations in both PCOS subjects and controls.[6] In addition, obese women with PCOS had lower HDL cholesterol and phospholipid concentrations in all subfractions compared with obese controls. This was in the presence of normal quantities of the protein component of HDL – apolipoprotein A1. These findings imply that the number of HDL particles was the same in obese PCOS subjects compared with obese controls, but the HDL particles were lipid-depleted and hence less effective in function. The only factor that appeared to have an independent influence on the HDL composition was the presence of PCOS, rather than obesity, or raised serum androgen or insulin concentrations.

Plasminogen activator inhibitor 1 (PAI-1) is a potent inhibitor of fibrinolysis and has been found to be elevated in both obese women and non-obese women with PCOS. Plasma levels of PAI-1 correlate directly with serum insulin concentrations and have been shown to be an important predictor of myocardial infarction.

Thus, the evidence is mounting that women with PCOS may have an increased risk of developing cardiovascular disease and diabetes later in life, which has important implications in their management.

## HYPERHOMOCYSTEINAEMIA

A moderately increased total plasma homocysteine concentration is associated with an increased risk of atherosclerosis. Homocysteine is an essential intermediate in the transfer of activated methyl groups from tetrahydrofolate to S-adenylmethionine, in the synthesis of cysteine from methionine and in the production of homocysteine thiolactone. An abnormal elevation of homocysteine in plasma and urine is caused by an imbalance between homocysteine production and metabolism, which can be of demographic, genetic, nutritional or metabolic aetiology and is associated with premature vascular disease. Mild hyperhomocysteinaemia has been demonstrated to induce sustained injury to the arterial endothelial cell, which accelerates the development of thrombosis and atherosclerosis. Normal concentrations of total plasma homocysteine are in the range of 5–16 μmol/l, although 10 μmol/l is considered the desired upper limit; there is an age-related rise and lower concentrations in women.

There have been reports of elevated plasma homocysteine in PCOS, although all studies were carried out predominantly on white European women. One report was the first to demonstrate an ethnic difference in the elevation of homocysteine in women with PCOS, which mirrors an ethnic variation in the degree of insulin resistance of PCOS.[7] Moreover, the significantly higher concentrations of plasma homocysteine and insulin among normal Sri Lankan women of reproductive age when compared with other control groups support the hypothesis of an inherent ethnic propensity to insulin resistance and hyperhomocysteinaemia among indigenous South Asians.

Randeva et al.[8] reported a significant decrease in plasma homocysteine and waist–hip ratio among young women with PCOS who are overweight or obese following six months of regular physical exercise. Weight reduction and regular physical exercise are recognised interventions that help towards reducing insulin resistance of the metabolic syndrome.

It is noteworthy that central obesity as determined by waist–hip ratio, an important component of the metabolic syndrome, showed a significant linear relationship with plasma homocysteine in PCOS. This is particularly significant in the light of Sri Lankan women with PCOS, who were found to have the highest mean concentration of homocysteine as well as the highest waist–hip ratio for a given BMI.[7] A difference in central obesity is also attributed to ethnic origin, with Asians being identified to have a higher body fat percentage at a lower BMI. These findings of the greatest severity in the cohort of young Sri Lankan women with PCOS who were recruited in an identical manner to the UK-based cohort recruitment are supported by the highest prevalence of glucose intolerance among Sri Lankan women with PCOS when compared with British Asians and white Europeans with PCOS. Nevertheless, the greater metabolic derangement observed in the indigenous Asians is likely to be explained by differing environmental influences.

## Polycystic ovary syndrome in younger women

At what stage do the risk factors for cardiovascular disease become apparent in women with PCOS? The majority of studies that have identified the risk factors of obesity and insulin resistance in women with PCOS have investigated adult populations, commonly including women who have presented to specialist endocrine or reproductive clinics. However, PCOS has been identified in much younger populations. A community-based study by Michelmore *et al.*[9] assessed the prevalence and associated features of polycystic ovaries in 230 young women aged 18–25 years. In this population, polycystic ovaries were identified in 33% and a high proportion of these women (80%) had one additional feature associated with PCOS. Of those with PCOS, 32% were overweight but none displayed a pattern of central obesity. Hyperinsulinaemia and insulin resistance were not identified in the women with polycystic ovaries, nor did they have elevated blood pressure. Women with increasing symptoms of PCOS, however, were found to be more insulin-resistant. These data emphasise the need for long-term prospective studies of young women with PCOS in order to clarify the natural history and to determine which women will be at risk of diabetes and cardiovascular disease later in life.

## Long-term follow-up in polycystic ovary syndrome

In 1992, Dahlgren *et al.*[4] extrapolated the findings of their earlier study to ascertain the relative risk of IHD in a group of 33 women diagnosed clinically and histologically to have PCOS between 1956 and 1965. By risk model analysis, it was calculated that the women with PCOS had a 7.4-fold greater risk of myocardial infarction than age-matched controls. Compared with the control group, the women with PCOS aged 40 years or older showed a marked increase in the prevalence of central obesity, higher basal serum insulin concentrations and a seven-fold higher prevalence of diabetes and three-fold higher prevalence of hypertension. However, in another study, Pierpoint et al.[10] reported the mortality rate in 1028 women diagnosed as having PCOS between 1930 and 1979. All the women were older than 45 years and 770 women had been treated by wedge resection of the ovaries; 786 women were traced: the mean age at diagnosis was 26.4 years and average duration of follow-up was 30 years. There were 59 deaths, of which 15 were from circulatory disease; 13 of these 15 deaths were from IHD. There were six deaths from diabetes as an underlying or contributory cause, compared with the expected 1.7 deaths. The standard mortality rate, both overall and for cardiovascular disease, was no higher in the women with PCOS when compared with the national mortality rates in women, although the observed proportion of women with diabetes as a contributory or under-lying factor leading to death was significantly higher than expected (OR 3.6, 95% CI 1.5–8.4). Thus, despite surrogate markers for cardiovascular disease, in this study no increased rate of death from cardiovascular disease could be demonstrated.

In a follow-up study by the same investigative group of 345 of these women with polycystic ovaries and 1060 age-matched controls there was no increased long-term coronary heart disease mortality in the group with polycystic ovaries, although there was evidence of increased stroke-related mortality, even after adjustment for BMI.[11]

## Therapeutic options

Obesity and insulin resistance, both together and in isolation, play a major role in increasing the risk of cardiovascular disease in women. Exercise and weight loss have so far been the most physiological way to improve insulin sensitivity and improve the metabolic abnormalities associated with the syndrome. In women with PCOS it has been demonstrated that even partial weight loss improves the hormonal profile and the reproductive outcome for all forms of fertility treatment. Since the association between insulin resistance and BMI is stronger in obese women with PCOS than in weight-matched controls, the benefits of weight loss should be even greater in these women than in women without PCOS.

There have been reports in the literature regarding the use of insulin-sensitising agents such as metformin and thiazolidinediones (troglitazone and rosiglitazone) in women with PCOS to reduce insulin resistance and improve the metabolic profile. Although troglitazone has been withdrawn from clinical use because of hepatotoxicity, metformin has shown some benefit. Most studied has been metformin, which may reduce insulin concentrations and improves insulin resistance. Some studies to date have demonstrated improvements in endocrine profiles, menstrual cyclicity and a reduction in PAI-1, together with an improvement in lipid profile, with varying degrees of and sometimes no weight loss. There is no consensus on dose or predictors for response and long-term follow-up studies are required.

# Polycystic ovary syndrome and cancer

The long-term risk of endometrial hyperplasia and endometrial carcinoma due to chronic anovulation and unopposed estrogen has long been recognised. Similarly, there may be an increased risk of breast carcinoma. The multifactorial nature of the syndrome, combined with its hetero-geneous presentation, makes it difficult to ascertain which factors (i.e. hyperinsulinaemia, elevated serum concentrations of growth factors, obesity or genetic predisposition) cause the most significant risk with respect to the development of cancer.

### ENDOMETRIAL CANCER

Although endometrial adenocarcinoma is the second most common female genital malignancy, only 4% of cases occur in women under 40 years of age. The risk of developing endometrial cancer has been shown to be adversely influenced by a number of factors, including obesity, long-term use of unopposed estrogens, nulliparity and infertility. In fact, the relative risk of endometrial cancer is 1.6 in women with a menarche before the age of 12 years and 2.4 in women with their menopause after the age of 52 years.[12] Women with endometrial carcinoma have fewer births compared with controls and it has also been demonstrated that infertility *per se* gives a relative risk of 2.0. Hypertension and type 2 diabetes have long been linked to endometrial cancer, with relative risks of 2.1 and 2.8, respectively[12] – these conditions are now known also to be associated with PCOS.

A study by Coulam *et al.*[13] examined the risk of developing endometrial carcinoma in a group of 1270 women who were diagnosed as having 'chronic anovulation syndrome'. The defining characteristics of this group included pathological or macroscopic evidence of the Stein–Leventhal syndrome, or a clinical diagnosis of chronic anovulation. This study identified the excess risk of endometrial cancer to be 3.1 (95% CI 1.1–7.3) and proposed that this might be due to abnormal levels of unopposed

## OVARIAN CANCER

There has been much debate about the risk of ovarian cancer in women with infertility, particularly in relation with the use of drugs to induce superovulation for assisted conception procedures. Inherently the risk of ovarian cancer appears to be increased in women who have multiple ovulations – that is, those who are nulliparous (possibly because of infertility) with an early menarche and late menopause. Thus, it may be that inducing multiple ovulations in women with infertility will increase their risk[22] – a notion that is by no means proven. Women with PCOS who are oligo-/anovulatory might therefore be expected to be at low risk of developing ovarian cancer if it is the lifetime number of ovulations rather than pregnancies that is critical. Ovulation induction to correct anovulatory infertility aims to induce unifollicular ovulation and so in theory should raise the risk of a woman with PCOS to that of a normal ovulating woman. The polycystic ovary, however, is notoriously sensitive to stimulation and it is only with the development of high-resolution transvaginal ultrasonography that the rate of unifollicular ovulation has attained acceptable levels. The use of clomifene citrate and gonadotrophin therapy for ovulation induction in the 1960s, 1970s and 1980s resulted in many more multiple ovulations (and indeed multiple pregnancies) than in more recent times and might therefore present with an increased rate of ovarian cancer when these women reach the age of greatest risk.

There are a few studies that have addressed the possibility of an association between polycystic ovaries and ovarian cancer. The results are conflicting and the potential for generalisation is limited due to problems with the study designs. In the large UK study of Pierpoint et al.,[10] the standardised mortality rate for ovarian cancer was 0.39 (95% CI 0.01–2.17).

# References

1 Lapidus L. Ischaemic heart disease, stroke and total mortality in women; results from a prospective population study in Gothenberg, Sweden. *Acta Med Scand Supp* 1986;**705**:1–42.

2 Reaven GM. Role of insulin resistance in human disease. *Diabetes* 1988;**37**:1595–607.

3 Burghen GA, Givens JR, Kitabchi AE. Correlation of hyperandrogenism with hyperinsulinism in polycystic ovarian disease. *J Clin Endocrinol Med* 1980;**50**:113–16.

4 Dahlgren E, Johansson S, Lindstedt G, Knutsson F, Oden A, Janson PO, *et al.* Women with polycystic ovary syndrome wedge resected in 1956 to 1965: a long term follow up focussing on natural history and circulating hormones. *Fertil Steril* 1992;**57**:505–13.

5 Gjonnaess H. The course and outcome of pregnancy after ovarian electrocautery in women with polycystic ovarian syndrome: the influence of

body-weight. *Br J Obstet Gynaecol* 1989;**96**:714–19.

6  Rajkhowa M, Neary RH, Knmptala P, Game FL, Jones P, Obhrai MS, *et al.* Altered composition of high density lipoproteins in women with the polycystic ovary syndrome. *J Clin Endocrinol Metab* 1997;**82**:3389–94.

7.  Wijeyaratne CN, Pathmakumara A, Warnakulasuriya AM, Gunawardhare AUA, Nirantharakunar K, Balen AH. Plasma homocysteine in polycystic ovary syndrome: does it correlate with insulin resistance and ethnicity? *Clin Endocrinol* 2004;**60**:560–67.

8.  Randeva HS, Lewandowski KC, Drzewoski J, Brooke-Wavell K, O'Callaghan C, Czupryniak L, *et al.* Exercise decreases plasma total homocysteine in overweight young women with polycystic ovary syndrome. *J Clin Endocrinol Metab* 2002;**87**:4496–501.

9  Michelmore K, Balen AH, Dunger D, Vessey M. Polycystic ovaries and associated clinical and biochemical features in young women. *Clin Endocrinol* 1998;**70**:S250.

10 Pierpoint T, McKeigue PM, Isaacs AJ, Wild SH, Jacobs HS. Mortality of women with polycystic ovary syndrome at long-term follow-up. *J Clin Epidemiol* 1999;**51**:779–86.

11 Wild S, Pierpoint T, McKeigue P, Jacobs H. Cardiovascular disease in women with polycystic ovary syndrome at long-term follow-up: a retrospective cohort study. *Clin Endocrinol* 2000;**52**:595–600.

12 Elwood JM, Cole P, Rothman KJ, Kaplan SD. Epidemiology of endometrial cancer. *J Natl Cancer Inst* 1977;**59**:1055–60.

13 Coulam CB, Annegers JF, Kranz JS. Chronic anovulation syndrome and associated neoplasia. *Obstet Gynecol* 1983;**61**:403–7.

14 Chamlian DL, Taylor HB. Endometrial hyperplasia in young women. *Obstet Gynecol* 1970;**36**:659–66.

15 Balen AH. Polycystic ovary syndrome and cancer. *Hum Reprod Update* 2001;**7**:522–5.

16 Ota T, Yoshida M, Kimura M, Kinoshita K. Clinicopathologic study of uterine endometrial carcinoma in young women aged 40 years or younger. *Int J Gynecol Cancer* 2005;**15**:657–62.

17 Niwa K, Tagami K, Lian Z. Outcome of fertility-preserving treatment in young women with endometrial carcinomas. *BJOG* 2005;**112**:317–20.

18 Yang YC, Wu CC, Chen CP, Chang CL, Wang KL. Reevaluating the safety of fertility-sparing hormonal therapy for early endometrial cancer. *Gynecol Oncol* 2005;**99**:287–93.

19 Jadoul P, Donnez J. Conservative treatment may be beneficial for young women with atypical endometrial hyperplasia or endometrial adeno-carcinoma. *Fertil Steril* 2003;**80**:1315–24.

20 Evans-Matcalf ER, Brooks SE, Reale FR. Profile of women 45 years of age and younger with endometrial cancer. *Obstet Gynecol* 1998;**91**:349–54.

21 Rackow BW, Arici A. Endometrial cancer and infertility. *Curr Opin Obstet Gynecol* 2006;**18**:245–52.

22 Nugent D, Salha O, Balen AH, Rutherford AJ. Ovarian neoplasia and subfertility treatments. *Br J Obstet Gynaecol* 1998;**105**:584–91.

# 10 Anovulatory infertility and ovulation induction

The principles of the management of anovulatory infertility are:

- to correct any underlying disorder (e.g. hypogonadotrophic women who are underweight)
- to optimise health before starting therapy (e.g. women with PCOS who are overweight)
- to induce regular unifollicular ovulation.

A semen analysis should be performed on the male partner before ovulation induction therapy is started. Tubal patency should be assessed by either hysterosalpingo-graphy or laparoscopy before embarking upon gonadotrophin therapy. If there are no firm indications (e.g. past history of pelvic infection, pelvic pain), a reasonable policy is to delay a test of tubal patency until there have been up to three or six ovulatory cycles. A complete assessment of every couple should be performed before choosing the appropriate therapy for inducing ovulation.[1]

## Pituitary and hypothalamic causes of anovulation

Anovulation may occur after surgery for pituitary tumours (Figure 10.1), pituitary ablation, Kallmann syndrome and hypogonadotrophic hypogonadism.

### HYPOGONADOTROPHIC HYPOGONADISM

If in the presence of estrogen deficiency the gonadotrophin concentrations are subnormal (less than 5 iu/l), hypogonadotrophic hypogonadism should be suspected. The cause may be at the level of the pituitary or hypothalamus. It used to be thought that stimulation with GnRH distinguished between a hypothalamic and pituitary aetiology. However, there is great heterogeneity in the response to a single 100-μg dose of GnRH in women with both hypothalamic and pituitary causes of anovulation. The GnRH test is therefore no longer performed. The diagnosis of Kallman syndrome is made if the woman has hyposmia

**Figure 10.1** Pituitary tumour; magnetic resonance imaging

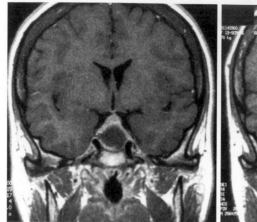
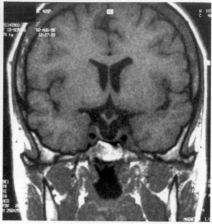

(a) before treatment with
   bromocriptine

(b) after treatment with
   bromocriptine, demonstrating the
   pituitary stalk

associated with hypogonadotrophic hypogonadism. Radiology of the hypothalamus and pituitary is otherwise indicated with either CT or MRI.

Ovulation is optimally induced in women with intact pituitary function by application of pulsatile luteinising hormone-releasing hormone (LHRH) or GnRH, administered subcutaneously or intravenously by a miniaturised infusion pump. The injections are given at intervals of 90 minutes at a dose of either 15 μg subcutaneously or 5–10 μg intravenously. This therapy provides the most physiological correction of the primary disturbance with little risk of multiple pregnancy or ovarian hyperstimulation. Ultrasound monitoring can be kept to a minimum and cumulative conception and livebirth rates equal those expected of normal ovulating women (Figure 10.2).

If pulsatile GnRH cannot be used (if the woman is unhappy with the equipment or if a pump is not available), then women with hypogonadotrophic hypogonadism of whatever cause respond better to hMG than to purified FSH, because the former contains the LH that is necessary to stimulate androgen steroidogenesis – the substrate for estrogen biosynthesis. Gonadotrophin therapy is described on pages 122–3.

## WEIGHT-RELATED AMENORRHOEA

A BMI of less than 20 kg/m² is subnormal. It is also necessary to achieve a BMI of more than 19 kg/m² before menarche (see Chapter 7). Although

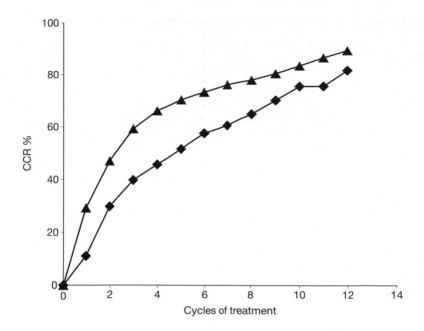

**Figure 10.2** Cumulative conceptions (CCR) over successive cycles in normal women (▲) and 77 with hypogonadotrophic hypogonadism (♦) who have undergone ovulation induction[6]

it may be easy to induce ovulation in these patients, they have an increased risk of obstetric problems (intrauterine growth restriction, stillbirth, neonatal death) and weight gain is therefore the correct therapy.

## Polycystic ovary syndrome (see also Chapter 8)

The management of anovulatory infertility in PCOS has traditionally involved the use of clomifene citrate and then gonadotrophin therapy or laparoscopic ovarian surgery in those who are clomiphene-resistant. There is no clear role for insulin-sensitising and insulin-lowering drugs, and algorithms for their place in therapy are still to be agreed upon. Newer therapeutic approaches include aromatase inhibitors and the potential use of *in vitro* maturation (IVM) of oocytes collected from unstimulated (or minimally stimulated) polycystic ovaries. There has been an unfortunate shift away from monofollicular ovulation induction to the use of in vitro fertilisation (IVF) treatment, based on a false premise of greater cumulative conception rates and appropriate concerns about multiple pregnancy. Superovulation for IVF presents significant risks for women with polycystic ovaries, namely the potentially life-threatening complication of ovarian hyperstimulation syndrome (OHSS). Carefully conducted and monitored ovulation induction can achieve good cumulative conception rates and, furthermore, multiple pregnancy rates can be minimised with strict adherence to criteria that limit the number of follicles that are permitted to ovulate.

PCOS accounts for approximately 80% of women with anovulatory infertility. Various factors influence ovarian function. Fertility is adversely affected by an individual being overweight or having elevated serum concentrations of LH. The principles of therapy are first to optimise health before commencing therapy and then induce regular unifollicular ovulation, while minimising the risks of OHSS and multiple pregnancy. Weight loss in those who are overweight improves the endocrine profile, the likelihood of ovulation and a healthy pregnancy and the response to every type of ovulation induction therapy.

Strategies to induce ovulation include first weight loss and then drugs to induce ovulation, with conventional first-line therapy being oral anti-estrogens (principally clomifene citrate), parenteral gonadotrophin therapy and laparoscopic ovarian surgery. There have been no adequately powered randomised studies to determine which of these therapies provides the best overall chance of a viable pregnancy as first line of therapy.

Appropriate pretreatment investigations are required, including a semen analysis of the male partner and an assessment of tubal patency. There are some who consider the latter unnecessarily invasive in those who are at low risk of tubal damage. It is considered, however, that it is important to exclude tubal damage before committing to the time and risks associated with ovarian stimulation.

Normal ovarian function relies upon the selection of a follicle, which responds to an appropriate signal (FSH) to grow, become 'dominant' and ovulate. This mechanism is disturbed in women with PCOS, resulting in multiple small cysts, most of which contain potentially viable oocytes but within dysfunctional follicles. Hypersecretion of LH is found in 40% of women with PCOS and is associated with a reduced chance of conception and an increased risk of miscarriage, possibly through an adverse effect of LH on oocyte maturation. The finding of a persistently elevated early to midfollicular phase LH concentration in a woman who is trying to conceive suggests the need to suppress LH levels by either pituitary desensitisation with a gonadotrophin-releasing hormone agonist or laparoscopic ovarian diathermy. There are, however, no large prospective randomised trials that demonstrate a therapeutic benefit from a reduction in serum LH concentrations during ovulation induction protocols. The assessment of serum LH concentration in the midfollicular stage of the stimulated cycle is helpful in predicting the likelihood of a successful outcome – particularly in the context of clomifene citrate therapy.

## LIFESTYLE AND WEIGHT LOSS IN POLYCYSTIC OVARY SYNDROME

The woman's BMI correlates with both hyperinsulinaemia and an increased rate of cycle disturbance and infertility. The greater the interval between menstrual periods, the greater the disturbance in insulin metabolism. Even moderate obesity, such as a BMI greater than 27 kg/m², is associated with a reduced chance of spontaneous ovulation or response to ovulation induction therapy. A body fat distribution leading to an increased waist–hip ratio appears to have a more detrimental effect than body weight alone, because of the metabolic activity of visceral fat. Monitoring treatment is also harder in women who are obese because their ovaries are more difficult to see on ultrasound scan, thus raising the risk of missing multiple ovulation and multiple pregnancy. National guidelines in the UK for managing women with PCOS who are overweight advise weight loss, preferably to a BMI less than 30 kg/m², before commencing drugs for ovarian stimulation.[2]

Clark et al.[3] studied the effect of a weight loss and exercise programme on women with a BMI greater than 30 kg/m² and anovulatory infertility who were clomifene citrate-resistant. The emphasis of the study was a realistic exercise schedule combined with positive reinforcement of a suitable eating programme over six months. Thirteen of the 18 women enrolled completed the study, reinforcing the difficulties some individuals have in sustaining even moderate changes in lifestyle. Weight loss had a significant effect on endocrine function, ovulation and the chance of pregnancy. Fasting insulin and serum testosterone concentrations fell and 12 of the 13 subjects resumed ovulation; 11 became pregnant – five spontaneously – and the remainder were now responsive to clomifene.

Thus, with appropriate support, women with PCOS may ovulate spontaneously without medical therapy. Even a modest loss of 5% of total body weight can achieve a reduction of central fat, an improvement in insulin sensitivity and restoration of ovulation. Lifestyle modification is clearly a key component for the improvement of reproductive function in overweight women with anovulation and PCOS.

The considerable risks in pregnancy associated with obesity are not usually appreciated when women with PCOS attend clinics and request fertility treatment.[4] It is well known that pregnancy carries considerable risks for women who are obese, including increased rates of congenital anomalies (neural tube and cardiac defects), miscarriage, gestational diabetes, hypertension and problems during delivery.[5,6] In addition, women with PCOS and obesity have an increased risk of gestational diabetes because of the additional insulin resistance caused by pregnancy itself. Increasingly, many women with PCOS have type 2 diabetes mellitus before conception. The outcomes of pregnancy in women with diabetes are much worse than in the general population and are at least equivalent to, if not slightly worse than, in women with type 1 diabetes.[7] Overweight mothers are also more likely than others to have hypertension and thromboembolism, leading to a higher risk of maternal mortality.[8] It is suggested that women with obesity and PCOS should try to attain a BMI of less than 30 kg/m² before starting ovulation induction and should even defer treatment with metformin until they reach a target BMI of 35 kg/m² or less. Consideration of age is important, but ultimately the main consideration should be for the potential health of the pregnant woman and any children born.

## CLOMIFENE CITRATE THERAPY

Anti-estrogen therapy with clomifene citrate has traditionally been used as first-line therapy for anovulatory PCOS. Clomifene citrate has been available for many years and its use has tended not to have been closely monitored. There have been no prospective randomised studies comparing the efficacy of clomifene with other therapies.[9] Anti-estrogen therapy is usually commenced on day two of the cycle and given for five days. If the woman has oligo-/amenorrhea it is necessary to exclude pregnancy and then induce a withdrawal bleed with a short course of a progestogen, such as medroxyprogesterone acetate 5–20 mg/day for five to ten days. The starting dose of clomifene is 50 mg/day for five days, beginning on days three to five of the menstrual cycle (the first day of bleeding is considered day one of the cycle). If the woman has not menstruated by day 35 and she is not pregnant, a progestogen-induced withdrawal bleed should be initiated. The dose of clomifene should only be increased if there is no response after three cycles as, of those women who will respond to 50 mg/day, only two-thirds will do so in the first cycle. Doses of 150 mg/day or more appear not to be of benefit. If there is an over-response to 50 mg/day, as in some women with PCOS, the dose can be decreased to 25 mg/day. Discontinuation of clomifene therapy should be considered if the woman is anovulatory after the dose has been increased up to 100 mg/day. If the woman is ovulating, conception is expected to occur at a rate determined by factors such as her age.

Clomifene may cause an exaggeration in the hypersecretion of LH and have anti-estrogenic effects on the endometrium and cervical mucus. All women who are prescribed clomifene should be monitored carefully with a combination of endocrine and ultrasonographic assessment of follicular growth and ovulation because of the risk of multiple pregnancies, which is approximately 10%. Clomifene therapy should therefore be prescribed and managed by specialists in reproductive medicine.

An ovulatory trigger in the form of parenteral administration of hCG is rarely required and should be given only if there has been repeated evidence of an unruptured follicle, by ultrasound and serum progesterone monitoring. Women with PCOS should have LH measured on day eight in a cycle that follows an ovulatory cycle; if the LH is greater than 10 iu/l, the chance of conception is reduced and risk of miscarriage is elevated. In this case, the options include laparoscopic ovarian diathermy and gonadotrophin therapy.

Clomifene induces ovulation in approximately 70–85% of women, although only 40–50% conceive. It is recommended that at least the first cycle of treatment, if not all cycles, should be monitored with a combination of serial ultrasound scans and serum endocrinology. Kousta et al.[10] reported treatment of 167 women with clomifene in whom there was a cumulative conception rate of 67.3% over six months in women who had no other subfertility factors, which continued to rise up to 12 cycles of therapy. These investigators reported a multiple pregnancy rate of 11.0%, similar to that described in other series and a miscarriage rate of 23.6%, with those who miscarried tending to have a higher serum LH concentration immediately after clomifene administration. If a pregnancy has not occurred after 10–12 normal ovulatory cycles, it is then appropriate to offer the couple assisted conception.

Women with anovulatory infertility who are resistant to anti-estrogens may be prescribed metformin combined with clomifene, parenteral gonadotrophin therapy or laparoscopic ovarian surgery. The term 'clomifene resistance' strictly speaking refers to a failure to ovulate rather than failure to conceive despite ovulation, which should be termed 'clomifene failure'.

## AROMATASE INHIBITORS

Aromatase inhibitors have been proposed as an alternative treatment to clomifene therapy, as the discrepancy between ovulation and pregnancy rates with clomifene has been attributed to its anti-estrogenic action and estrogen receptor depletion. The aromatase inhibitors suppress estrogen production and thereby mimic the central reduction of negative feedback through which clomifene works. Letrozole, the most widely used anti-aromatase for this indication, has been shown to be effective, in early trials, in inducing ovulation and pregnancy in women with anovulatory PCOS and inadequate clomifene response and improving ovarian response to FSH in poor responders. Anastrozole is currently being examined as a possible alternative. Evidence from larger trials is still awaited but some encouragement may be taken from the solidity of the working hypothesis and the success of the preliminary results. The role of aromatase inhibitors in an algorithm for ovulation induction has yet to be agreed. Furthermore, the possible teratogenicity of aromatase inhibitors has to be fully evaluated and manufacturers currently do not advise their use for ovulation induction.

## GONADOTROPHIN THERAPY

Gonadotrophin therapy is indicated for women with anovulatory PCOS who have been treated with anti-estrogens and who have either failed to ovulate or, if they responded to clomifene, developed other issues reducing their chance of conception (such as persistent hypersecretion of LH).

To prevent the risks of overstimulation and multiple pregnancy with gonadotrophin therapy, the traditional standard step-up regimens (when 75–150 iu/day is increased by 75 iu/day every 3–5 days) have been replaced by either 'low-dose step-up' regimens or 'low-dose step-down' regimens.

The low-dose step-up regimen employs a starting daily dose of 0.50–0.75 of an ampoule (37.5–50.00 iu/day), which is only increased after 14 days if there is no response and then only by half an ampoule every seven days. Treatment cycles using this approach can be quite long (up to 28–35 days) but the risk of multiple follicular growth is lower than with conventional step-up regimens. The initiation of follicular growth requires a 10–30% increment in the dose of exogenous FSH and the threshold changes with follicular growth, because of an increased number of FSH receptors, so that the concentration of FSH required to maintain growth is less than that required to initiate it. In ovulation induction protocols, stimulation with gonadotrophins does not require a background of pituitary desensitisation. To date, there is no difference in efficacy between the different gonadotrophin preparations.

It can be challenging to stimulate the development of a single dominant follicle in women with PCOS. Although attempts have been made to predict a multifollicular response by determining midfollicular endocrine profiles and numbers of small follicles, it is harder to do so before starting ovarian stimulation and hence to determine the required starting dose of gonadotrophin. To prevent multiple pregnancy, strict criteria are required before the administration of hCG with no more than two follicles greater than 14 mm, with the largest greater than 17 mm. White et al.[11] reported their extensive experience of the low-dose regimen in 225 women over 934 cycles of treatment and resulting in 109 pregnancies in 102 women (45%). Seventy-two percent of the cycles were ovulatory (less than 5% of women failed to ovulate) and 77% of these uniovulatory. The multiple pregnancy rate was 6%. Despite using a low-dose protocol, 18% of cycles were abandoned because more than three large follicles developed: a further reminder of the sensitivity of the polycystic ovary even when attempts are made to reduce the response. The only factor that influenced the outcome significantly was the woman's BMI: those women with a BMI greater than 25 kg/m$^2$ had a higher rate of abandoned cycles (31% compared with 15% in those of normal weight), a lower cumulative conception rate over six cycles (46.8% compared with 57% for the whole group) and a miscarriage rate of 31%. Another series reported the cumulative conception and livebirth rates in 103 women with clomifene-resistant PCOS;[12] the cumulative conception and livebirth rates after six months were 62% and 54%, respectively and, after 12 months, 73% and 62%, respectively.

## SURGICAL OVULATION INDUCTION

An alternative to gonadotrophin therapy for clomifene-resistant PCOS is laparoscopic ovarian surgery, which has replaced the more invasive and damaging technique of ovarian wedge resection. Laparoscopic ovarian surgery is free of the risks of multiple pregnancy and ovarian hyperstimulation and does not require intensive ultrasound monitoring. Furthermore, laparoscopic ovarian diathermy (LOD) appears to be as effective as routine gonadotrophin therapy in the treatment of clomifene-insensitive PCOS.[13] In addition, laparoscopic ovarian surgery is a useful therapy for anovulatory women with PCOS who fail to respond to clomifene and who persistently hypersecrete LH, who need a laparoscopic assessment of their pelvis or who live too far away from the hospital to be able to attend for the intensive monitoring required of gonadotrophin therapy. Surgery carries its own risks and must be performed only by fully trained laparoscopic surgeons.

After laparoscopic ovarian surgery, with restoration of ovarian activity, serum concentrations of LH and testosterone fall. Whether women respond to LOD appears to depend on their pretreatment characteristics, with women who have high basal LH concentrations having a better clinical and endocrine response. A small prospective study[14] randomised women to receiving either unilateral or bilateral LOD and found that unilateral diathermy restored bilateral ovarian activity, with the contralateral, untreated ovary often being the first to ovulate after the diathermy treatment. The only significant difference between the responders and nonresponders was a post-diathermy fall in serum LH concentration.

Commonly employed methods for laparoscopic surgery include mono-polar electrocautery (diathermy) and laser, while multiple biopsy alone is less commonly used. The greater the amount of damage to the surface of the ovary, the greater the risk of periovarian adhesion formation. This led to the development of a strategy of minimising the number of diathermy points to four per ovary for 4 seconds at 40 watts. Wedge resection of the ovaries resulted in significant adhesions, in 100% of cases in some published series. The risk of adhesion formation is far less after laparoscopic ovarian diathermy (10–20% of cases) and the adhesions that do form are usually fine and of limited clinical significance. It is advisable to instil 1000 ml icodextrin 4% in electrolytes (Adept®, ML Laboratories) solution into the pouch of Douglas, which, by cooling the ovaries, prevents heat injury to adjacent tissues and reduces the adhesion formation.

Ovarian diathermy appears to be as effective as routine gonadotrophin therapy in the treatment of clomifene-insensitive PCOS. The Cochrane database concludes that, although there is insufficient evidence to demonstrate a difference between 6 and 12 months of follow-up after LOD and three to six cycles of ovulation induction with gonadotrophins, multiple pregnancy rates are considerably reduced with LOD.[12] The largest randomised controlled trial to date is the multicentre study performed in The Netherlands, in which 168 women resistant to clomifene were randomised to either LOD ($n$ = 83) or ovulation induction with recombinant FSH (rFSH, $n$ = 65).[15] The initial cumulative pregnancy rate after six months was 34% in the LOD arm compared with 67% with rFSH. Those who did not ovulate in response to LOD were then given first clomifene and then rFSH and so, by 12 months, the cumulative pregnancy rate was similar in each group at 67%.[15] Thus, those treated with LOD took longer to conceive and 54% required additional medical ovulation induction therapy.

It has been suggested that, to demonstrate a 20% increase in pregnancy rate over six months from 50% to 70%, with an 80% power, at least 235 women would be required in each arm of a study to compare LOD with gonadotrophin therapy. The current meta-analysis in the Cochrane database includes a total of only 303 women.[13] The continuing pregnancy rate following ovarian drilling compared with gonadotrophins differed according to the length of follow-up. Overall, the pooled odds ratio for all studies was not statistically significant (OR 1.27, 95% CI 0.77–1.98). Multiple pregnancy rates were reduced in the ovarian drilling arms of the four trials where there was a direct comparison with gonadotrophin therapy (OR 0.16, 95% CI 0.03–0.98). There was no difference in miscarriage rates in the drilling group when compared with gonadotrophin in these trials (OR 0.61, 95% CI 0.17–2.16).

## THE ROLE OF METFORMIN AND OTHER INSULIN SENSITISERS

It is logical to assume that therapy achieving a fall in serum insulin concentrations should improve the symptoms of PCOS. The biguanide metformin both inhibits the production of hepatic glucose, thereby decreasing insulin secretion, and enhances insulin sensitivity at the cellular level. The efficacy of metformin in PCOS was first described by Velazquez et al.[16] and many studies have been carried out to evaluate the reproductive effects of metformin in women with PCOS. Most of the initial studies, however, were observational and any randomised studies published involved a small number of participants. Indeed, two systematic reviews revealed that the majority of the published studies on the effects of metformin alone on the menstrual cycle in women with PCOS had a sample size of less than 30 women.[17,18]

Metformin ameliorates hyperandrogenism and abnormalities of gonadotrophin secretion in women with PCOS and can also restore menstrual cyclicity. Metformin appears to be less effective in those who are significantly obese (BMI greater than 35 kg/m²) and there are still no agreed algorithms for its use. Furthermore, there is no agreement on predictors for response or the appropriate dose and whether dose should be adjusted for body weight or other factors.

Initial studies appeared to be promising, suggesting that metformin could improve fertility in women with PCOS. However, more recent large randomised controlled trials (RCTs) have observed that the beneficial effects of metformin first-line therapy for the treatment of the anovulatory woman with PCOS is significantly less than clomifene. In a multicentre trial of 20 Dutch hospitals, 228 women with with PCOS were treated either with clomifene plus metformin or clomifene plus placebo.[19] The ovulation rate in the metformin group was 64%, compared with 72% in the placebo group, a nonsignificant difference. There were no significant differences in either rate of continuing pregnancy (40% compared with 46%) or rate of miscarriage (12% compared with 11%). A significantly larger proportion of women in the metformin group discontinued treatment because of adverse effects (16% compared with 5%). The investigators concluded that metformin was not an effective addition to clomifene as the primary method of inducing ovulation in women with PCOS.

A preliminary report of the Pregnancy in Polycystic Ovary Syndrome (PPCOS) trial, sponsored by the US National Institutes of Health (NIH), noted that metformin alone was significantly less effective than clomifene alone as first-line therapy for the treatment of anovulatory women with PCOS who are infertile and that the addition of metformin to clomifene produces only marginal benefits.[20] This multicentre study enrolled 676 infertile women with PCOS (diagnosed by an elevated testosterone levels and oligomenorrhea with eight or more spontaneous menses/year, after exclusion of secondary causes of hyperandrogenemia) who were seeking pregnancy. All were not taking confounding medications and were in otherwise good health, were aged 18–39 years and had no other obvious infertility factors, with at least one patent fallopian tube, normal uterine cavity and a partner with a sperm concentration of 20 million/ml in at least one ejaculate. After progestin withdrawal, these women were equally randomised to three different treatment arms for a total of six cycles or 30 weeks:

- metformin 1000 mg twice daily plus placebo
- clomifene 50 mg every day for five days (days three to seven of cycle) plus placebo
- combined metformin 1000 mg twice daily plus clomifene 50 mg/day for five days (days three to seven).

Overall, livebirth rates were 7.2% (5/208), 22.5% (47/209) and 26.8% (56/209), respectively, with the metformin alone group being significantly lower than the other two groups. Pregnancy loss rates tended to also be higher in the metformin alone group (40.0% compared with 22.6% and 25.5%, respectively).[20]

The combined effects of lifestyle modification and metformin on anovulatory women who were obese (BMI greater than 30 kg/m$^2$) and had PCOS were studied in a prospective randomised, double blind, placebo-controlled multicentre trial.[20] All the women had an individualised assess-ment by a research dietitian to set a realistic goal that could be sustained for a long period of time, with an average reduction of energy intake of 500 kcal/day. As a result, both the metformin-treated and placebo groups managed to lose weight but the amount of weight reduction did not differ between the two groups. An increase in menstrual cyclicity was observed in those who lost weight but again did not differ between the two arms of the study.[21]

The variable findings from published studies on the use of metformin reflect the large differences in study populations, particularly with respect to body weight. Insulin sensitivity decreases (or insulin resistance increases) with BMI. It has been known that women with PCOS who are not obese respond better to metformin than do women who are obese.[22,23] Mmetformin may have a direct effect on ovarian function and enhances the outcome of some fertility therapies in some women – probably those with relatively mild metabolic dysfunction. There has been a tendency to discontinue metformin once a pregnancy has been achieved, although a number of studies have confirmed its apparent safety, with lack of teratogenicity and potential for reducing the risk of miscarriage and gestational diabetes, although large RCTs are awaited.

The insulin-sensitising agent troglitazone also appeared to improve the metabolic and reproductive abnormalities in PCOS significantly, although this product has been withdrawn because of reports of fatal liver damage. The new generation of thiazolidinediones (rosiglitazone and pioglitazone) may be of benefit to the older woman with PCOS but should not be prescribed to women wishing to conceive because of an uncertain safety profile in pregnancy. Newer insulin-sensitising agents are currently being evaluated, as is the phosphoglycan-containing drug D-chiro-inositol.

# IVF IN WOMEN WITH POLYCYSTIC OVARIES

IVF is not the first line of treatment for PCOS but many women with the syndrome may be referred for IVF, either because there is another reason for their infertility or because they fail to conceive despite ovulating (whether spontaneously or with assistance); that is, their infertility remains unexplained. Furthermore, approximately 30% of women have polycystic ovaries as detected by ultrasound scan. Many will have few symptoms and may present for assisted conception treatment because of other reasons (for example, tubal factor or male factor). When stimulated, these women with asymptomatic polycystic ovaries have a tendency to respond sensitively and are at increased risk of developing OHSS.

The response of the polycystic ovary to stimulation in the context of ovulation induction aimed at the development of unifollicular ovulation is well documented and differs significantly from that of normal ovaries. The response tends to be slow, with a significant risk of ovarian hyperstimulation. Conventional IVF depends on inducing multifollicular recruitment and, again, the response of the polycystic ovary differs from the normal, with a potentially 'explosive' response, based on the presence of many partially developed follicles present in the polycystic ovary. Thecal hyperplasia (in some cases with raised levels of LH and/or insulin) provides large amounts of androstenedione and testosterone, which act as substrates for estrogen production. Granulosa cell aromatase, although deficient in the 'resting' polycystic ovary, is readily stimulated by FSH. Therefore, normal quantities of FSH act on large amounts of substrate (testosterone and androstenedione) to produce large amounts of intra-ovarian estrogen. Ovarian follicles, of which there are too many in polycystic ovaries, are increasingly sensitive to FSH (receptors for which are stimulated by high local concentrations of androgens and estrogen) and, as a result, there is multiple follicular development associated with very high levels of circulating estrogen. In some cases, this may result in OHSS, to which women with polycystic ovaries are particularly prone.

In addition, insulin acts as a co-gonadotrophin and augments theca cell production of androgens in response to stimulation by LH and granulosa cell production of estrogen in response to stimulation by FSH. There is also widespread expression of vascular endothelial growth factor (VEGF) in polycystic ovaries. VEGF is an endothelial cell mitogen that stimulates vascular permeability, hence its involvement in the pathophysiology of OHSS. VEGF is normally confined in the ovary to the blood vessels and is responsible there for invasion of the relatively avascular graafian follicle by blood vessels after ovulation. The increase of LH at midcycle leads to expression of VEGF, which has been shown to be an obligatory intermediate in the formation of the corpus luteum. It has been shown that, compared with women with normal ovaries, women with polycystic ovaries or PCOS have increased serum VEGF.

The above data serve to remind us of the close relationship of polycystic ovaries with OHSS and also provide a possible explanation for the multifollicular response of the polycystic ovary to gonadotrophin stimulation. One of the mechanisms that underpins the unifollicular response of the normal ovary is diversion of blood flow within the ovaries, first from the nondominant to the dominant ovary and, second, from cohort follicles to the dominant follicle. This results in diversion of FSH away from the cohort follicles and permits them to undergo atresia. The widespread distribution of VEGF in polycystic ovaries may prevent this diversion of blood flow, leaving a substantial number of small and intermediate-sized follicles in 'suspended animation' and ready to respond to gonadotrophin stimulation. The distribution of VEGF in the polycystic ovary therefore helps to explain one of the fundamental features of the polycystic ovary, namely the loss of the intraovarian autoregulatory mechanism that permits unifollicular ovulation to occur.

Case–control studies of the outcome of IVF in women with polycystic ovaries compared with controls who have normal ovaries have consistently shown the development of more follicles, higher serum estradiol concentrations and more eggs but often lower fertilisation rates. Rates of OHSS are significantly higher than controls at 10% compared with the expected rate of 1%.

A long-running debate in ovulation induction for women with PCOS is whether the use of FSH alone has any benefit over hMG – is the hypersecretion of LH responsible for the exaggerated response to stimulation of the polycystic ovary? Does minimising circulating LH levels by giving FSH alone improve outcome? The consensus from a combination of meta-analyses suggests that there is no difference in outcome whether hMG, urinary FSH or recombinant FSH is used.[24,25]

The introduction of schedules of gonadotrophin stimulation that incorporate treatment with GnRH antagonists holds promise for women with polycystic ovaries and PCOS. GnRH antagonists do not activate the GnRH receptors and produce a rapid suppression of gonadotrophin secretion within hours. A Cochrane systematic review showed that there is a trend of reduction of ovarian hyperstimulation syndrome in the GnRH antagonist treatment groups with the combined odds ratio of 0.47 (95% CI 0.18–1.25).[26] A dramatic reduction in the rate of OHSS has also been shown with the use of metformin for the first four weeks of an IVF treatment cycle.[21]

## *IN VITRO* MATURATION OF OOCYTES

In recent years, IVM has attracted interest as a new assisted reproductive technique. The immature oocytes are retrieved from antral follicles of unstimulated (or minimally stimulated) ovaries via the transvaginal approach. The oocytes are subsequently matured *in vitro* in a special formulated culture medium for 24–48 hours. The mature oocytes are fertilised, usually by intracytoplasmic sperm injection (ICSI), and the selected embryos are transferred to the uterus two or three days later. Although IVM is labour-intensive compared with conventional IVF treatment, there are a number of clinical advantages by the avoidance of large doses of exogenous gonadotrophins, most importantly by avoiding the risk of OHSS. Since women with PCOS have more antral follicles and a higher risk of developing OHSS compared with those without PCOS, IVM may be a promising alternative to conventional IVF.

Significantly more immature oocytes are retrieved from polycystic ovaries than from normal ovaries and the overall oocyte maturation and fertilisation rates are similar among the three groups. The subsequent pregnancy and livebirth rates for transfer are then significantly higher in women with polycystic ovaries because of a greater choice in the embryos selected for transfer. IVM yields significantly fewer mature oocytes than IVF cycles and therefore fewer embryos per retrieval. Implantation rates are still lower in IVM compared with IVF cycles, which may be due to a reduced oocyte potential or a reduced endometrial receptivity.[27] It is hoped that continuous improvements in the culture medium and synchrony between endometrial and embryonic development will result in better IVM success rates in the future.

## Risks of ovulation induction

Multiple pregnancy is an undesirable adverse effect of fertility therapy because of the increased rates of perinatal morbidity and mortality. In the UK, it is the unmonitored use of oral antiestrogens that accounts for more cases of triplets than do gonadotrophin therapy or assisted conception.

High-order multiple pregnancies (quadruplets or more) result almost exclusively from ovulation induction therapies. Gonadotrophins should be given in low doses to women with anovulatory infertility and strict criteria should be used before the administration of the ovulatory trigger.

If conception has failed to occur after six ovulatory cycles in a woman younger than 25 years, or after 12 ovulatory cycles in a woman older than 25 years, then it can be assumed that anovulation is unlikely to be the cause of the couple's infertility. Assisted conception (usually IVF) is now indicated.

## Ovarian hyperstimulation syndrome

The pathophysiological hallmark of OHSS is a sudden increase of vascular permeability that results in the development of a massive extravascular exudate. This exudate accumulates primarily in the peritoneal cavity, causing a protein-rich ascites. Loss of fluid into the 'third' space causes a profound fall in intravascular volume, haemoconcentration and suppression of urine formation. Loss of protein into the third space causes a fall in plasma oncotic pressure that results in further loss of intravascular fluid. Secondary hyperaldosteronism occurs and causes salt retention. Eventually peripheral oedema develops.

| CLASSIFICATION OF OHSS | |
|---|---|
| **Grade 1 (mild)** | Characterised by fluid accumulation, as evidenced by weight gain, and abdominal distension and discomfort. Ultrasound examination shows enlarged ovaries with a diameter greater than 5 cm. |
| **Grade 2 (moderate)** | Associated with the development of nausea and vomiting; the ovarian enlargement and abdominal distension are greater and cause more discomfort and dyspnoea. Ascites can be detected by ultrasound. |
| **Grade 3 (severe)** | A life-threatening condition in which there is clinical evidence of contraction of the intravascular volume (subnormal central venous pressure with reduced cardiac output), severe expansion of the third space (tense ascites, pleural and pericardial effusions, all of which compromise the circulation and breathing), severe haemoconcentration and the development of hepatorenal failure. In addition to the circulatory crisis, these patients are at risk from intravascular thrombosis. |

Deaths have been recorded in women with grade 3 OHSS, caused usually by cerebrovascular thrombosis, renal failure or cardiac tamponade resulting from pericardial effusion. OHSS usually occurs only after overstimulated ovaries have been exposed to hCG. The condition therefore results most commonly when sensitive (i.e. polycystic) ovaries are exposed to excessive quantities of FSH and then to hCG. The finding that severe OHSS is often associated with pregnancy is probably related to the persistence of hCG in this situation. Even when the ovaries have been severely overstimulated, OHSS can always be prevented by avoiding exposure of the ovaries to LH and/or hCG.

Most methods of ovarian stimulation can cause OHSS. The overall risk is estimated to be about 4% and that of the severe form about 0.25%. Severe cases occur in 0.25–2.0% of IVF cycles.

## MANAGEMENT OF OVARIAN HYPERSTIMULATION SYNDROME

Mild ovarian hyperstimulation is managed expectantly,[27] its importance being that it should alert both patient and doctor to the risk of a more severe condition developing. The patient should be encouraged to take abundant fluids. A marked increase in weight (more than 5 kg) combined with developing abdominal distension, nausea and vomiting indicate the onset of grade-2 hyperstimulation and a need for hospitalisation. In non-conception cycles, moderate ovarian hyperstimulation can be expected to resolve with the development of menstruation, although the ovarian cysts may persist for a month or so more.

Women with grade-2 OHSS need careful assessment. Oral fluids are encouraged, although vomiting may make an intravenous infusion necessary. If luteal support is required, progesterone and not hCG should be used. Full-length thromboembolism deterrent stockings are recommended to reduce the risk of deep-vein thrombosis and prophylactic enoxaparin 20 mg should be given daily. Adequate analgesia is required. Preferred drugs are paracetamol, with or without codeine, and pethidine for severe pain.

The development of clinically detectable and usually painful ascites, together with deterioration in respiration, circulation and renal function, indicates the development of severe grade-3 hyperstimulation and, in most cases, the need for admission to an intensive care unit. The intravascular volume should be monitored by measurements of central venous pressure (CVP), renal function by meticulous attention to input and urine output and haemoconcentration by measurement of haematocrit, whose level reflects intravascular volume depletion and blood viscosity. A haematocrit of over 45% is a serious warning sign and a measurement greater than 55% signals a life-threatening situation. There may be a striking leucocytosis, the white blood cell count rising up to 40 000 ml. Measurement of body weight, serum urea, creatinine and electrolytes, together with serum albumin and liver function tests and periodic assessments of the coagulation profile, are mandatory.

Infusion of colloid is required to maintain intravascular volume, as indicated by restoration of normal CVP. The choice lies between human albumin (50–100 g repeated as required) or intravenous dextran or hydroxyethyl starch, although the latter compounds carry the risk of anaphylactic reaction and dextran has been implicated in severe acute respiratory distress syndrome. Crystalloid (usually physiological saline) is administered for rehydration. If urine flow remains suppressed despite restoration of CVP and rehydration, abdominal paracentesis should be undertaken under ultrasound guidance. The indications for this procedure are therefore the need for symptomatic relief of a tense ascites, oliguria, rising serum creatinine, falling creatinine clearance and haemoconcentration unresponsive to medical therapy. Severe oliguria or renal failure persisting despite these measures usually necessitates dialysis.

Paracentesis of hydrothorax should be considered for relief of dyspnoea. Cardiac tamponade from pericardial effusion may prove fatal if not rapidly relieved. Careful cardiological assessment together with cardiac ultrasound should therefore feature in the management of these patients. The possibility of reaccumulation of fluid in any of these cavities should be considered.

Surgery should be avoided in patients with OHSS, except if there is evidence of ovarian torsion or marked haemorrhage or rupture of one of the ovarian cysts. Diuretics are contraindicated in these patients. Anticoagulation (subcutaneous heparin in a dose of 5000 iu twice daily) is indicated if there is evidence of thromboembolism or a deteriorating coagulation profile.

## Summary

The key principle in achieving ovulation induction for women with PCOS is to achieve unifollicular ovulation and thereby avoid the significant risks of multiple pregnancy and OHSS. Clomifene citrate still remains the first-line medical therapy for anovulatory PCOS. It may be time to rethink current strategies, particularly with the promising early experience of metformin. Furthermore, studies are under way comparing gonadotrophin therapy with clomifene as first-line treatment.

Compared with medical ovulation induction with gonadotropins for the woman who is clomifene-resistant, the advantage of LOD is that it need be performed only once and intensive monitoring is not required, as there is no danger of multiple ovulation or ovarian hyperstimulation. Gonadotrophin therapy appears to provide similar long-term cumulative conception rates as LOD, although time to pregnancy is quicker. In the future, gonadotrophin therapy may be made easier by the use of long-acting FSH preparations and orally active agents.

| OVULATION INDUCTION KEY POINTS |
| :-- |

- Correction of the cause of anovulatory infertility will lead to cumulative conception rates that approach those expected for the woman's age.
- It is important to optimise health, confirm tubal patency and check the partner's semen analysis before starting treatment.
- Hypogonadotrophic hypogonadism is best treated by pulsatile GnRH but if gonadotrophins are required use hMG rather than FSH.
- PCOS should be treated first with clomifene citrate. If this fails, gonadotrophin therapy and laparoscopic ovarian diathermy are efficacious, with the latter being associated with lower multiple pregnancy rates.
- Clomifene citrate therapy should be carefully monitored; doses greater than 100 mg confer no benefit and, if ovulation is occurring, it is reasonable to continue for at least 6 but no more than 12 months.
- Gonadotrophin therapy requires close monitoring with serial ultrasound scans, the main risks being multiple pregnancy and OHSS.
- Laparoscopic ovarian diathermy is a single treatment that works well in selected patients.
- Metformin has not proved to be of significant benefit, particularly in those who are overweight.

# References

1 Balen AH, Jacobs HS. *Infertility in Practice.* 2nd ed. London: Churchill Livingstone; 2003.

2 National Collaborating Centre for Women's and Children's Health. *Fertility: Assessment and Treatment for People with Fertility Problems.* London: RCOG Press; 2004.

3 Clark AM, Ledger W, Galletly C, Tomlinson L, Blaney F, Wang X, *et al.* Weight loss results in significant improvement in pregnancy and ovulation rates in anovulatory obese women. *Hum Reprod* 1995;**10**:2705–12.

4 Balen AH, Dresner M, Scott EM, Drife JO. Should obese women with polycystic ovary syndrome (PCOS) receive treatment for infertility? *BMJ* 2006:**332**:434–5.

5 Cedergren MI. Maternal morbid obesity and the risk of adverse pregnancy outcome. *Obstet Gynecol* 2004;**103**:219–24.

6 Linné Y. Effects of obesity on women's reproduction and complications during pregnancy. *Obes Rev* 2004;**5**:137–43.

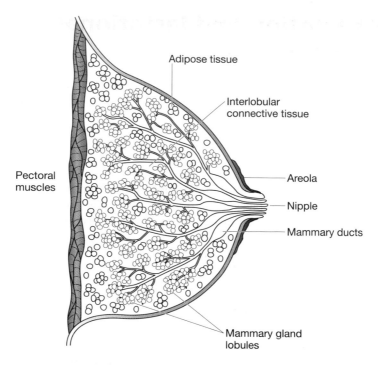

**Figure 11.1** Structure of the breast during lactation

milk production. Prolactin concentrations thus remain high during lactation, declining eventually as the frequency of feeding lessens.

Delivery of milk from the alveolar cells to the infant's mouth is achieved by contraction of the surrounding myoepithelial cells, which is stimulated by oxytocin, secreted in a pulsatile fashion from the posterior pituitary.[2] Oxytocin secretion itself starts in response to afferent stimuli from the nipple, caused by suckling. In the early puerperium, the uterus still contains numerous oxytocin receptors and suckling may be accompanied by 'after-pains' (uterine contractions), particularly in multiparous women.

In the absence of feeding, or after cessation of regular suckling, falling levels of prolactin result in the slowing of milk production. Eventually, unused milk is reabsorbed and the alveolar cells regress, returning the breast architecture to a similar (though not identical) state to that of the nulliparous breast.

Psychological stimuli, particularly stress, may affect oxytocin production; a commonly observed phenomenon is letdown of milk in response to hearing the crying of an infant. The opposite may also occur and stress may be responsible for inhibition of oxytocin production and resultant failure of breastfeeding.

# Endocrine effects of lactation

## AMENORRHOEA

Lactation leads to ovarian quiescence, which results in amenorrhoea. This occurs in response to the almost complete cessation of pituitary gonadotrophin release, centrally mediated via a loss of the pulsatile secretion of GnRH from the hypothalamus. The exact cause of this remains unclear. Although an obvious explanation would appear to be the high levels of prolactin associated with lactation, there is little direct evidence for this and the mechanism appears to be via a more complex central pathway. It has been shown that the normal positive feedback response of the anterior pituitary to estrogens is lost during lactation, thus preventing ovulation from occurring even when estrogen levels rise.

The most important initiator of a return to normal fertility appears to be the introduction of supplementary artificial feeds via a bottle to a previously exclusively breastfed baby, heralding a decline in the frequency of the suckling stimulus. Research techniques involving serial ten-minute blood sampling of women in various stages of lactation have shown supplements are associated with the recommencement of pulses of LH.

## HYPOESTROGENAEMIA

Long-term amenorrhoea is a hypoestrogenic state and this can result in genital atrophy and vaginal dryness, causing pain and dyspareunia, particularly if there has been perineal trauma at the time of birth. This can be overcome by the use of lubricants for sexual activity and, if necessary, local estrogens. In longer-term lactational amenorrhoea, there have been concerns about the development of osteoporosis; however, it has been shown that bone mass is quickly regained following the return of ovarian activity.[3,4]

## SOCIAL EFFECTS

There has been interest for some years in the association between lactational hormones and improved interaction between mother and baby. Research in other mammals tends to suggest improved bonding attributable to oxytocin, although this is difficult to prove in humans.

# Metabolic effects of lactation

## DIET

The necessary dietary requirements of lactation have long been the subject of debate. There is clear evidence, especially in poorer parts of the world, that energy intakes of lactating women fall well below that expected when total calorie output, including that of the breast milk, is measured. The exact cause of this discrepancy is unclear, although a form of metabolic adaptation is implied. A diminution of basal energy expenditure has been demonstrated in lactating women and work in rats has suggested an overall increase in insulin sensitivity, although this has not been shown in humans.

## WEIGHT CHANGE

The pattern of weight loss following delivery is complex. It would appear that women who breastfeed have less postpartum weight retention than women who do not. Other factors such as maternal age are also important.

## CONTROL OF LACTATION

Drugs have been used for both the stimulation and the inhibition of lactation. There is no known condition where milk production is entirely absent and true deficiency is thought to be rare. Breastfeeding problems are usually associated with poor letdown, which can be caused by stress, poor feeding technique and separation from the baby. Oxytocin nasal sprays and metoclopramide to stimulate prolactin production have been tried for improvement in milk yield, with variable results. The need for such preparations is far outweighed by the simple application of good midwifery teaching on breastfeeding technique (particularly latching-on of the baby to the breast), permanent access to the baby where possible, the avoidance of supplementary artificial feeding and appropriate encouragement and reassurance.

Dopamine agonists such as bromocriptine and cabergoline, which result in a reduction in prolactin secretion, are effective at inhibiting lactation and formerly were used widely in women with healthy term babies who did not wish to breastfeed or in whom breast engorgement was a serious problem. Although dopamine agonists are still in use to ease breast symptoms following the loss of a baby, it is far better under normal circumstances to treat engorgement with frequent breastfeeds and with firm breast support if the woman is not breastfeeding.

# Lactation and contraception

## NATURAL CONTRACEPTION

The amenorrhoea resulting from lactation provides a form of contraception, the lactational amenorrhoea method (LAM). Provided that three rules are followed, the method is 98% effective and therefore comparable with modern artificial methods of family planning.[5]

## RULES FOR SUCCESSFUL USE OF THE LACTATIONAL AMENORRHOEA METHOD

- The baby must be under 6 months old.
- The mother must be amenorrhoeic.
- The mother must exclusively breastfeed the baby on demand day and night, remembering that even a small amount of supplementary artificial feeding may lead to a return in ovulation.

If used with appropriate education and good user motivation, LAM provides a safe method of preventing conception following recent childbirth, with avoidance of all the associated maternal hazards, physical and social, of one pregnancy following close upon another. As it is entirely natural, LAM should also be acceptable to religious groups opposed to artificial contraception. With the added advantages of being free, and associated with the safest and most effective method of providing infant nutrition, LAM is an obvious choice, particularly in developing countries, where health groups are actively encouraging its continued use.

## ARTIFICIAL CONTRACEPTION

Few women in Western societies rely solely on LAM. Suitable artificial contraceptives for lactating women are the progesterone-only pill, depot progestogens, barrier methods and the interval insertion of an intra-uterine contraceptive device. The combined pill is generally not recommended because, theoretically, the estrogen component may lead to inhibition of lactation and it may be secreted in breast milk. These concerns are probably unfounded with modern low-estrogen pills but, in view of the reduced natural fertility during lactation, there is less need for such an effective contraceptive.

## LACTATION KEY POINTS

- Lactation is initiated and controlled by a variety of endocrine mechanisms.
- Although breast milk confers a number of advantages on both baby and mother, the most important immediate effect of lactation for the mother is amenorrhoea and reduced fertility resulting from gonadotrophin downregulation.
- Pharmacological manipulation of lactation is no substitute for good midwifery.

# References

1 Glasier A, McNeilly A. Physiology of lactation. *Baillieres Clin Endocrinol Metab* 1990;**4**:379–95.

2 Buhimschi CS. Endocrinology of lactation. *Obstet Gynecol Clinic North Am* 2004;**31**:963–79, xii.

3 Hadji P, Ziller V, Kalder M, Gottschalk M, Hellmeyer L, Hars O, *et al.* Influence of pregnancy and breast-feeding on quantitative ultrasonometry of bone in postmenopausal women. *Climacteric* 2002;**5**:277–85.

4 More C, Bettembuk P, Bhattoa HP, Balogh A. The effects of pregnancy and lactation on bone mineral density. *Osteoporosis Int* 2001;**12**:732–7.

5 World Health Organization Task Force on Methods for the Natural Regulation of Fertility. Lactational amenorrhea. I. Description of infant feeding patterns and of the return of menses. *Fertil Steril* 1998;**70**:448–60.

# 12 Hyperprolactinaemia

Hyperprolactinaemia is the most common pituitary cause of amenorrhoea. There are many causes of a mildly elevated serum prolactin concentration, including stress and a recent physical or breast examination. If the prolactin concentration is greater than 1000 milliunits per litre (mu/l), then the test should be repeated and, if still elevated, it is necessary to image the pituitary fossa with a CT or MRI scan (Figure 12.1). Hyperprolactinaemia may result from a prolactin-secreting pituitary adenoma or from a nonfunctioning 'disconnection' tumour in the region of the hypothalamus or pituitary, which disrupts the inhibitory influence of dopamine on prolactin secretion. Large nonfunctioning tumours are usually associated with serum prolactin concentrations of less than 3000 mu/l, while prolactin-secreting macroadenomas usually result in concentrations of 8000 mu/l or more. Other causes include hypothyroidism, PCOS (up to 2500 mu/l) and several drugs (e.g. the dopaminergic antagonist phenothiazines, domperidone and metoclopramide).

In women with amenorrhoea associated with hyperprolactinaemia, the main symptoms are usually those of estrogen deficiency. In contrast, when hyperprolactinaemia is associated with PCOS, the syndrome is characterised by adequate estrogenisation, polycystic ovaries on ultrasound scan and a withdrawal bleed in response to a progestogen challenge test. Galactorrhoea may be found in up to one-third of women with hyper-prolactinaemia, although its appearance is correlated neither with prolactin levels nor with the presence of a tumour. Approximately 5% of patients present with visual field defects.

A prolactin-secreting pituitary microadenoma (Figure 12.1) is usually associated with a moderately elevated prolactin (1500–4000 mu/l) and is unlikely to result in abnormalities on a lateral skull X-ray. On the other hand, a macroadenoma (Figure 12.2a,b) associated with a prolactin concentration greater than 5000–8000 mu/l, and by definition greater than 1 cm in diameter, may cause typical radiological changes – that is, an asymmetrically enlarged pituitary fossa, with a double contour to its floor and erosion of the clinoid processes. CT and MRI scans allow detailed examination of the extent of the tumour and, in particular, identification of suprasellar extension and compression of the opitic chiasma or invasion

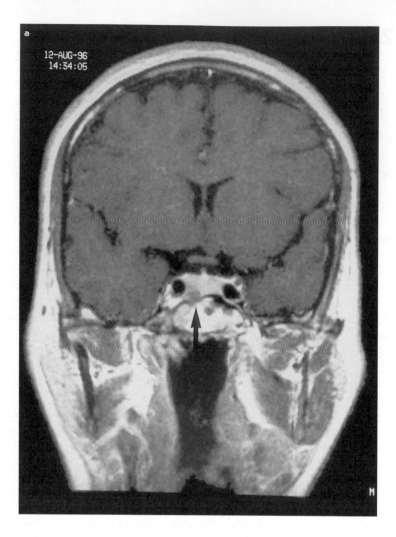

**Figure 12.1** Pituitary microadenoma: cranial magnetic resonance imaging; a coronal section T1-weighted spin echo sequence after intravenous gadolinium; the normal pituitary gland is hyperintense (bright) while the tumour is seen as a 4-mm area of non-enhancement (grey) in the right lobe of the pituitary, encroaching up to the right cavernous sinus; it is eroding the right side of the sella floor (arrow); reproduced with permission of Churchill Livingstone from Balen and Jacobs, *Infertility in Practice*, 2003

of the cavernous sinuses (there is no longer a place for plain X-ray in the diagnostic work-up of hyperprolactinaemia). Prolactin is an excellent tumour marker and therefore the higher the serum concentration, the

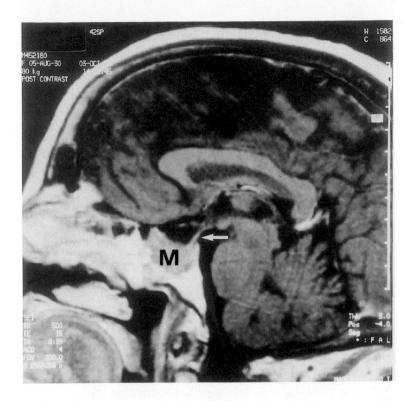

**Figure 12.2a** Pituitary macroadenoma: cranial magnetic resonance imaging coronal section at level of the pituitary stalk (arrow). The macroadenoma (M) is expanding from the left lobe of the pituitary gland into the left cavernous sinus and is bulging superiorly to deviate the pituitary stalk towards the right

larger the size of the tumour expected on the MRI scan. In contrast, a large tumour on the scan with only a moderately elevated serum prolactin concentration (2000–3000 mu/l) suggests a nonfunctioning tumour with 'disconnection' from the hypothalamus (Figure 12.3a,b).

## MEDICAL MANAGEMENT

The management of hyperprolactinaemia centres around the use of a dopamine agonist, of which bromocriptine is the most widely used . If the hyperprolactinaemia is drug-induced, stopping the relevant preparation should, of course, be recommended. This may not, however, be appropriate if the cause is a psychotropic medication, for example a phenothiazine being used to treat schizophrenia. In these cases, it is

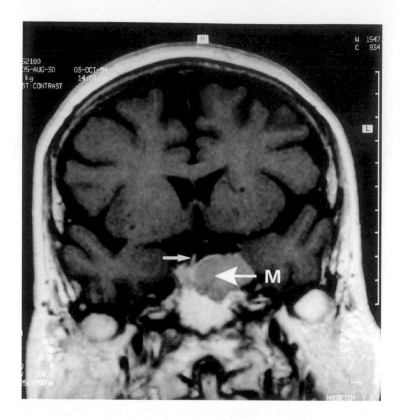

**Figure 12.2b** Magnetic resonance imaging of a pituitary macroadenoma: T1-weighted image post-gadolinium enhancement demonstrating a macroadenoma with a large central cystic component (large arrow); there is suprasellar extension with compression of the optic chiasm (small arrow)

reasonable to continue the drug and prescribe a low-dose combined oral contraceptive preparation in order to counteract the symptoms of estrogen deficiency. Serum prolactin concentrations must then be monitored carefully to ensure that they do not rise further.[1]

Most women show a fall in prolactin levels within a few days of commencing bromocriptine therapy and a reduction of tumour volume within six weeks. Adverse effects can be troublesome (nausea, vomiting, headache, postural hypotension) and are minimised by starting the therapy at night for the first three days of treatment and taking the tablets in the middle of a mouthful of food. Longer-term adverse effects include Raynaud's syndrome, constipation and psychiatric changes – especially aggression, which can occur at the start of treatment.

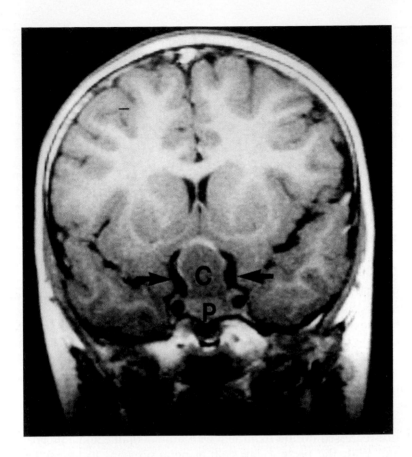

**Figure 12.3a** Magnetic resonance imaging of a craniopharyngioma: coronal T1-weighted section after gadolinium enhancement; the tumour signal intensity on the T1 image and only part of the periphery of the tumour enhances; the carotid arteries have a low signal intensity (black arrows) due to the rapid flow within them and are deviated laterally and superiorly by the mass (C), which arises out of the pituitary fossa (P)

Bromocriptine should be started at a dose of half a tablet at night (1.25 mg) and increased gradually, every 5 days until a dose of 2.5 mg at night is reached then 1.25 mg in the morning together with the 2.5 mg at night increased until the daily dose is 7.5 mg (in two or three divided doses). The maintenance dose should be the lowest that works and is often lower than that needed initially to initiate a response.

Longer-acting preparations (e.g. quinagolide, twice-weekly cabergoline) may be prescribed to those women who develop unacceptable adverse

| Table 12.1 | Drug therapy for hyperprolactinaemia | |
|---|---|---|
| Drug | Dose | Maintenance |
| Bromocriptine | 2.5–20 mg daily, divided doses | 5.0–7.5 mg/day |
| Cabergoline | 0.25–1 mg twice weekly | 1 mg/day |
| Quinagolide | 25–150 µg daily, divided doses | 75 µg/day |

effects. Cabergoline generally appears to be better tolerated and more efficacious than bromocriptine. The longer-acting preparations may be associated with psychiatric adverse effects and so therapy commences with bromocriptine (Table 12.1). Furthermore, cabergoline is not licensed for use in early pregnancy.

## SURGICAL MANAGEMENT

Surgery, in the form of a transsphenoidal adenectomy, is reserved for cases of drug resistance and failure to shrink a macroadenoma or where there are intolerable adverse effects of the drugs (the most common indication). Non-functioning tumours should be removed surgically and are usually detected by a combination of imaging and a serum prolactin concentration of less than 3000 mu/l. When the prolactin level is 3000–8000 mu/l, a trial of bromocriptine is warranted and if the prolactin level falls it can be assumed that the tumour is a prolactin-secreting macroadenoma. Operative treatment is also required if there is suprasellar extension of the tumour that has not regressed during treatment with bromocriptine and a pregnancy is desired. With the present-day skills of neurosurgeons in transsphenoidal surgery, it is seldom necessary to resort to pituitary irradiation, which offers no advantages, and long-term surveillance is required to detect consequent hypopituitarism (which is immediately apparent if it occurs after surgery).

## EFFECT ON PREGNANCY

Women with a microprolactinoma who wish to conceive can be reassured that they may stop bromocriptine when pregnancy is diagnosed and require no further monitoring, as the likelihood of significant tumour expansion is less than 2%. On the other hand, if a woman with a macroprolactinoma is not treated with bromocriptine, the tumour has a 25% risk of expanding during pregnancy. This risk is probably also present if the tumour has been treated but has not shrunk, as assessed by CT or MRI scan. The first-line approach to treatment of macroprolactinomas is therefore with bromocriptine combined with barrier methods of contraception. In cases with suprasellar expansion, follow-up CT (or MRI)

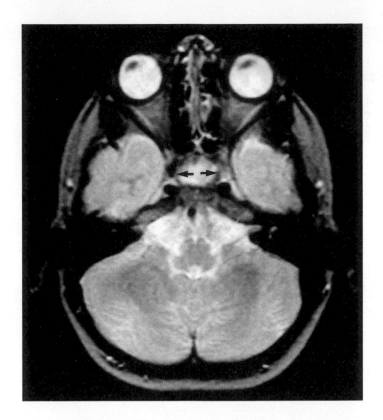

**Figure 12.3b** Cranial magnetic resonance imaging of a craniopharyngioma: axial T-weighted section, without enhancement, made just above the level of the pituitary gland and through the chiasmatic cistern; there is a high signal in the suprasellar extension of the tumour (arrowed); reproduced with permission of Churchill Livingstone from Balen and Jacobs, *Infertility in Practice*, 2003

should be performed after three months of treatment to ensure tumour regression, before it is safe to embark upon pregnancy. Bromocriptine can be discontinued during pregnancy, although if symptoms suggestive of tumour re-expansion occur an MRI scan should be performed and if there is continuing suprasellar expansion it is necessary to recommence bromocriptine therapy. These patients also require expert assessment of their visual fields during pregnancy, every two to three months.

If the serum prolactin is found to be elevated and the woman has a regular menstrual cycle, no treatment is necessary unless the cycle is anovulatory and fertility is desired. Amenorrhoea is the 'bioassay' of prolactin excess and should be corrected for its sequelae, rather than for the serum level of prolactin.

## Reference

1 Soule SG, Jacobs HS. Prolactinomas: present day management. *Br J Obstet Gynaecol* 1995;**102**:178–81.

# 13 Thyroid disease

Thyroid disease is more common in women than men. Hypothyroidism occurs in 2.0% of women at some stage in their lifetime, and hyperthyroidism occurs in about 2.5% of women. Thyroid disease is frequently subclinical and a high index of suspicion is thus required. Thyroid function tests may be part of the normal work-up in a number of clinical scenarios, such as menstrual disorders, pubertal problems, osteoporosis, infertility and possibly recurrent miscarriage. Thyroid replacement hormones are never indicated with normal thyroid function tests as a way of enhancing weight loss or boosting fertility.

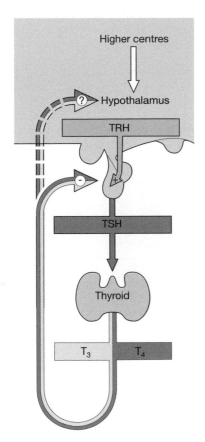

## Scientific background

The thyroid gland produces thyroxine ($T_4$) and triiodothyronine ($T_3$). An adequate dietary supply of iodine is needed for normal thyroid hormone production. The iodine is absorbed as iodide by the small intestine and transported to the thyroid gland. The uptake of iodide by the thyroid is under the influence of thyroid-stimulating hormone (TSH). TSH is a dimeric glycoprotein that has the same

**Figure 13.1** Schematic representation of the hypothalamic–pituitary–thyroid axis; $T_3$, triiodothyronine; $T_4$, thyroxine; TRH, thyrotropin-releasing hormones; TSH, thyroid-stimulating hormone

alpha subunit as FSH, LH and hCG but has a unique beta subunit. Normal secretion of the thyroid hormones is dependent upon TSH being released by the anterior pituitary gland (Figure 13.1).

The secretion of TSH is inhibited by the thyroid hormones and stimulated by the release of thyrotropin-releasing hormone (TRH) from the hypothalamus. Iodide in the serum is trapped by the thyroid cells and then oxidised and incorporated into some of the tyrosine residues of thyroglobulin. Monoiodotyrosine and diiodotyrosine combine to form $T_3$ and $T_4$. The thyroid gland contains stores of thyroglobulin in the lumen of the thyroid follicles, which is resorbed by the thyroid follicular cells, hydrolysed and released as $T_3$ and $T_4$ into the circulation. Thyroxine is secreted in much greater quantities than $T_3$ and one-third of $T_4$ is converted by peripheral tissues to $T_4$. $T_3$ is the more biologically active form, as it is less tightly protein-bound than $T_4$, resulting in ten times the concentration of free $T_3$ than $T_4$. The thyroid hormones in the blood are bound to serum-binding proteins, mostly thyroid-binding globulin (TBG), with small amounts also bound to prealbumin and albumin so that little circulates as free $T_3$ or free $T_4$ (less than 0.1%). It is the free hormone fraction that determines the action of the hormones in target tissues. $T_3$ forms when one iodine is removed from the phenolic ring of $T_4$; when an iodine from the nonphenolic ring is removed, reverse $T_3$ ($rT_3$) forms. Reverse $T_3$ is biologically inactive and one-third of the $T_4$ secreted daily is converted to $rT_3$ by peripheral tissues.

## Thyroid function

**Table 13.1   Drugs that may affect thyroid function tests**

| Drug | Mechanism |
| --- | --- |
| Oral contraceptive pill | ↑ binding proteins |
| Clomifene | ↑ binding proteins |
| Tamoxifen | ↑ binding proteins |
| Androgens | ↓ binding proteins |
| Glucocorticoids | ↓ binding proteins |
| Danazol | ↓ binding proteins |
| Iodine | ↓ $T_3$ and ↓ $T_4$ |
| Lithium | ↓ $T_3$ and ↓ $T_4$ |
| Cholestyramine | ↓ iodine absorption from the gut |
| Propylthiouracil | Inhibit $T_4$ to $T_3$ conversion |
| Amiodarone | Inhibit $T_4$ to $T_3$ conversion |

| THYROID FUNCTION TESTS (see also Tables 13.1 and 13.2) | |
|---|---|
| Thyroid-stimulating hormone (TSH) | Measured using a monoclonal antibody assay, which is highly sensitive. TSH concentration is the best guide to thyroid hormone production. Transient alterations in TSH levels may be caused by systemic illness such as psychiatric disease and drugs such as steroids. <br> Normal range 0.20–6.00 mu/l. |
| Free thyroxine ($T_4$) | A displacement assay measures $T_4$ using an antibody to $T_4$. <br> Normal range 12–27 nmol/l. |
| Total thyroxine | A displacement assay measures both free and bound thyroxine. In practice, free thyroxine is all that is needed. <br> Normal range 60–140 nmol/l. |
| Total triiodothyronine ($T_3$) | This may be measured using immunoassays but has little to add in clinical usefulness compared with the free thyroxine assay. <br> Normal range 1.0–2.5 nmol/l. |

## CLINICAL EXAMINATION OF THE THYROID GLAND

After observing the thyroid gland, palpation should be carried out by standing behind the patient. The thyroid gland should also be observed

**Table 13.2  Diagnosis of thyroid disorders according to thyroid function tests**

| Diagnosis | Serum free thyroxine | Serum-sensitive thyroid-stimulating hormone |
|---|---|---|
| Hypothyroidism | | |
|   Hypothyroidism | ↓ | ↑ |
|   Incipient hypothyroidism | Normal | ↑ |
|   Hypothalamic/pituitary hypothyroidism | ↓ | ↓ |
| Hyperthyroidism | | |
|   Hyperthyroidism | ↑ | Undetectable |
|   Incipient hyperthyroidism | Normal | ↓ |
|   Pituitary hyperthyroidism | ↑ | ↑ |

and palpated while the patient swallows a mouthful of water. A bruit may be auscultated over a goitre. The lymph nodes in the neck should also be examined. A thyroglossal cyst may be differentiated from a thyroid nodule in that the former moves upwards on protrusion of the tongue.

## Classification and diagnosis (Table 13.2)

### SIMPLE NON-TOXIC GOITRE

This is an enlargement of the thyroid gland that is not associated with abnormalities of thyroid function or with a neoplastic or inflammatory process. Simple non-toxic goitres may occur in areas of iodine deficiency, although often the cause is unknown. Usually there are no symptoms, unless the goitre becomes so large as to mechanically compress the trachea. The diagnosis may only be made in the presence of normal thyroid function tests and after cancer and an inflammatory process have been excluded. Treatment is required with thyroxine to lower the normal TSH levels and 'rest' the thyroid gland.

### HYPOTHYROIDISM

This is either primary, where the problem is at the level of the thyroid gland or, in rare cases, secondary to diminished TSH secretion. Hypothyroidism is thought to be due to an autoimmune problem and may be associated with other autoimmune diseases or a family history of thyroid disease. When a goitre is also present, hypothyroidism is termed Hashimoto's thyroiditis. A goitre should never be treated with thyroid hormones unless thyroid function tests are abnormal. Hypothyroidism is also associated with abnormal lipoprotein profile, which improves following treatment of the thyroid disorder.

**Clinical presentation**

---

**SYMPTOMS AND SIGNS OF HYPOTHYROIDISM**

**Symptoms**
Fatigue, cold intolerance, constipation, menstrual disturbance, depression
**Signs**
Goitre, dry skin, delayed reflexes, bradycardia, myxoedema, periorbital oedema

---

Menstrual problems ranging from amenorrhoea to menorrhagia may occur. Sometimes the serum prolactin concentration is elevated due to concomitant stimulation by an increase in TRH. Myxoedema is the accumulation of mucopolysaccharides in the dermis of the skin, causing a doughy induration of the skin and thickening of the facial features. Cretinism is hypothyroidism dating from birth and occurs in one in 5000 births. If not treated promptly, it leads to developmental delays, retarded bone age and characteristic facies. Thus, every neonate should be screened for hypothyroidism shortly after birth.

Thyroid function tests should also be performed in patients with pubertal problems and recurrent miscarriage and as part of the normal fertility work-up.

### Diagnosis
Raised TSH and lowered $T_3$ and $T_4$ (TSH may be normal or low in hypothalamic or pituitary hypothyroidism, which is rare).

### Management
Treat with daily thyroxine ($T_4$). The usual dose is 50–150 μg per day. However, the initial dose may need to be lower if there is any possibility of cardiac disease. The response to treatment is monitored clinically and by measuring TSH. The hypothalamic–pituitary axis takes eight weeks to recover and, thus, on stopping or altering medication, this length of time must elapse before re-evaluating TSH and $T_4$.

## HYPERTHYROIDISM

There are two main forms of hyperthyroidism: Graves' disease (toxic diffuse goitre) and toxic nodular goitre (Plummer's disease). Toxic nodular goitre usually arises in a longstanding goitre in postmenopausal women. Graves' disease is thought to be caused by autoantibodies that bind to the TSH receptors on the thyroid gland and activate them. Any nodule in the thyroid must be investigated in order to exclude possible malignancy using fine-needle aspiration, ultrasound and/or radioactive iodine uptake test.

### Clinical presentation
The thyroid gland is enlarged in 60% of patients with hyperthyroidism. Premenopausal women with hyperthyroidism frequently have eye signs that may consist of exophthalmos, lid lag and ophthalmoplegia. The course of the ocular disease often does not accompany that of the thyroid disease and may be difficult to treat. Specialised ophthalmic help is often required. Weight loss may occur despite a good appetite. Menstrual disturbances such as amenorrhoea or oligomenorrhoea may occur. In rare instances, hyperthyroidism may present in overt heart failure either with or without atrial fibrillation.

## SYMPTOMS AND SIGNS OF HYPERTHYROIDISM

**Symptoms**

Nervousness, gritty eyes, heat intolerance, frequent bowel movements, weight loss

**Signs**

Tachycardia, fine tremor, goitre, sweatiness, brisk reflexes, atrial fibrillation, eye signs, e.g. exophthalmos, lid lag, opthalmoplegia and watery eyes, hypotension, shock post-surgery, tachycardia, diabetes, cholelithiasis

### Diagnosis

Raised TSH, $T_3$ and $T_4$. Rarely, hyperthyroidism may be due to an excess of TSH production such as a pituitary tumour or a stimulating influence of trophoblastic origin (hCG) such as a hydatidiform mole or a choriocarcinoma.

### Management

There are a number of options available for the treatment of hyperthyroidism, including medication, surgery and radioactive ablative therapy. Medication such as propranolol (40–80 mg per day) may be used to control symptoms and drugs such as carbimazole and propylthiouracil to suppress hormone synthesis. The usual dose of carbimazole is 20–60 mg per day until the patient becomes euthyroid, and then it is reduced to a maintenance dose of 5–15 mg per day. The women should be warned about the rare complication of agranulocytosis associated with carbimazole. The usual dose of propylthiouracil is 100–150 mg every six to eight hours. If pregnancy is being contemplated, propylthiouracil is the preferred drug because of the potential low risks with carbimazole of aplasia cutis in the infant.

If drug therapy fails, an ablative procedure is usually carried out, with the long-term risk of hypothyroidism and consequent replacement therapy. Ablative therapy may be either radioactive iodine or a surgical subtotal thyroidectomy. Radioactive iodine is the therapy of choice for toxic nodular goitre.

### Hyperthyroidism and osteoporosis

Hyperthyroidism has been identified as another risk factor for osteoporosis as thyroid hormones increase bone resorption. Calcium levels are also increased, leading to a decrease in parathyroid hormone level that results in less vitamin D hydroxylation, which also increases bone resorption. Thus, physiologically appropriate thyroid hormone replacement therapy needs to be given, with monitoring of TSH levels.

## Pregnancy and the thyroid gland

During pregnancy, the TBG levels increase due to the hyperestrogenic effect on the liver but the pregnant woman remains euthyroid, with a normal TSH, free $T_3$ and $T_4$. This occurs by way of an increase in thyroid activity that is thought to be due to the effects of hCG and another chorionic thyrotropin from the placenta. Thus, a new equilibrium of free thyroid hormone is attained, with increase in the bound fraction. Many women with hyperemesis gravidarum have hyperthyroidism, which often resolves spontaneously when the vomiting settles. These thyroid abnormalities may be due to the increased levels of hCG observed in these women.

## Hyperthyroidism in pregnancy

Hyperthyroidism occurs in two in 1000 pregnancies and, if untreated, results in an increased risk of pre-eclampsia, fetal growth restriction, stillbirth and maternal heart failure due to the combined effects of hyperthyroidism and pregnancy. Ultrasound can usually exclude trophoblastic disease as the cause. Presentation may be with hyperemesis or failure to gain weight.

The signs of hyperthyroidism are difficult to separate from the normal hyperdynamic state of pregnancy and a laboratory diagnosis is needed. The laboratory diagnosis is not affected by pregnancy. Treatment is with drugs or surgery. Propylthiouracil is the favoured agent, as carbimazole crosses the placenta more easily. The dose should be kept as low as possible so as to avoid the possibility of hypothyroidism in the fetus and neonate, although no deleterious effects have been observed. Propylthiouracil does not conflict with breastfeeding, as it is so highly protein-bound that little passes into the milk.

When antibodies against the thyroid TSH receptor are present, these may cross the placenta and cause fetal thyrotoxicosis and death. Current tests for the antibodies are nonspecific. The fetus may be treated by treating the mother and assessing the neonatal thyroid state a few days postpartum. These antibodies may be present in women with Hashimoto's or Graves' disease even if the mother is now euthyroid or has undergone a thyroidectomy.

## Hypothyroidism

Women with severe hypothyroidism rarely become pregnant. Moderate hypothyroidism occurs in nine in 1000 pregnancies and is associated with pre-eclampsia, growth restriction and possibly miscarriage. The dose of thyroxine usually needs to be increased slightly during pregnancy using the maternal TSH level for monitoring.

## Postpartum thyroiditis

Four to eight percent of women experience this condition, which is thought to be due to a destructive thyroiditis associated with microsomal antibodies. Transient hyperthyroidism usually occurs followed by hypothyroidism and presents at three to six months postpartum, tending to last one to three months. Postpartum thyroiditis may present as postnatal depression and has also been implicated as a possible predisposing factor for postnatal depression. Thyroid function tests should be performed in women with postnatal depression. Postpartum thyroiditis is associated with autoimmune disease or previous postpartum thyroiditis. Women with this condition are at risk of hypothyroidism in later life.

## Fetal and neonatal thyroid physiology

The fetal thyroid gland begins to secrete $T_4$ at 10–13 weeks of gestation at the same time as the fetal pituitary begins to secrete TSH. At around 20 weeks, an increase in TSH and $T_4$ occurs. Fetal $T_4$ levels rise throughout pregnancy. Within 30 minutes of delivery, TSH levels peak, followed by a $T_3$ peak at 24 hours and a $T_4$ peak at 24–48 hours. Normal laboratory values are present by day four or five. These dramatic changes that occur at birth are thought to be triggered by exposure of the baby to a cold environment and may be an inbuilt protective mechanism.

## De Quervain's thyroiditis

This is a viral thyroiditis and often follows an upper respiratory chest infection. The thyroid gland is usually exquisitely tender and the erythrocyte sedimentation rate is raised. Treatment is with aspirin; in more severe cases, corticosteroids may be used.

---

**THYROID DISEASE KEY POINTS**

- TSH and free thyroxine measurements are the most clinically useful tests of thyroid function and it is rare for other tests to be required.
- Menstrual disorders may be a manifestation of thyroid disease, and thyroid function tests are indicated.
- Hyperthyroidism is a risk factor for osteoporosis.
- In pregnancy, the rise in TBG production is compensated by an increase in thyroid hormone production so that an equilibrium is maintained and thyroid function tests are within the normal range.

---

# 14 Diabetes

Diabetes mellitus is the term used for a group of heterogeneous disorders characterised by glucose intolerance and hyperglycaemia resulting either from excess glucose or the lack of effect of endogenous insulin. This metabolic condition results in changes in many aspects of bodily haemostasis but also has an effect on reproductive capability from conception, to pregnancy and childbirth. This chapter describes the pathophysiology of type 1, insulin-dependent diabetes mellitus, its treatment and control, the relevant aspects for fertility, pregnancy and management of gestational diabetes. There is further discussion of the relationship between type 2, non-insulin-dependent diabetes, insulin resistance, hyperinsulinaemia and PCOS (see also Chapter 9).

Banting and Best first described insulin in 1922. This revolutionised the management of type 1 diabetes, which had severe implications for pregnant women and their children. The perinatal mortality in diabetic pregnancy was at that time 440/1000 and it continued at that level for several decades until improvements in prepregnancy and antepartum control were made. Maternal and fetal morbidity and mortality have been greatly improved through the combined effects of a greater understanding of the disease, the use of more purified insulins with variable duration of effect and improved surveillance during pregnancy. In recognition of the variable but still excessive morbidity and mortality, the St Vincent declaration of 1989 set a five-year target for reduction of adverse pregnancy outcomes among women with type 1 diabetes to a level equivalent to that among women without diabites.

The physiological changes of pregnancy include increased glucose loading, hyperinsulinaemia and increased insulin resistance (especially in the third trimester). This results in high postprandial glucose levels and a tendency to lower fasting glucose levels. The latter may be due to an increase in maternal plasma volume and uteroplacental blood flow, thereby facilitating increased glucose extraction by the fetoplacental unit. The mechanism of insulin resistance may be related to increasing levels of human placental growth hormone (hPGH), human chorionic somatomammotrophin (hCS) and other diabetogenic hormones exerting effects on insulin action at a post-receptor level. Pancreatic islet cells

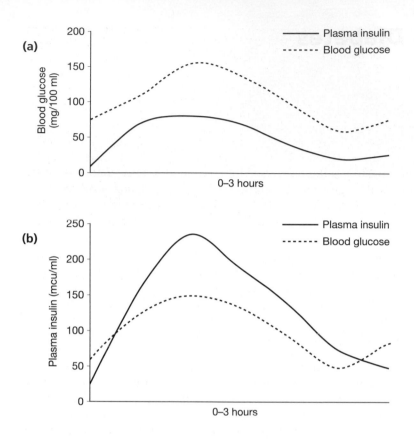

**Figure 14.1** The insulin secretion response to oral glucose (100 g) in (a) normal and (b) pregnant women

hypertrophy in response to this demand, an adaptation that is limited in diabetics. In gestational diabetes, hyperglycaemia and retarded glucose utilisation result in an increased glucose pool. The inability to mount an acute insulin response during a glucose challenge followed by a delayed but sustained secretion of insulin contrasts with that of the nonpregnant woman (Figure 14.1). After delivery, the rapid reversal of glucose intolerance in gestational diabetes is clinical evidence that fetoplacental factors are responsible for gestational diabetogenesis.

## Definition

World Health Organization definitions of impaired glucose tolerance and diabetes mellitus are based on a nonpregnant population (Table 14.1).[1] This would put 10% of the normal population in the impaired glucose

**Table 14.1** Glucose tolerance test (GTT) screening values for nonpregnant and pregnant women after a 75-g glucose load

| | GTT screening values | | |
|---|---|---|---|
| | Fasting | 1 hour | 2 hour |
| Impaired glucose tolerance | | | |
|   Nonpregnant population [a] | ≤ 7.8 mmol/l | | ≥ 7.8 and ≤ 11.0 mmol/l |
|   Pregnant population [b] | | ≥ 10.5 mmol/l | ≥ 9 and ≤ 11.0 mmol/l |
| Diabetes mellitus [a] | > 7.8 mmol/l | | >11 mmol/l |

[a] World Health Organization[1] criteria; [b] Lind[2] criteria

tolerance category. In pregnancy, other studies have proposed adjusting these thresholds such that gestational impaired glucose tolerance is diagnosed with a one-hour glucose of 10.5 mmol/l or more and a two-hour glucose of 9 mmol/l or more and 11 mmol/l or less.[2]

# Treatment and control

Insulin derived from the pancreatic beta cells of animals had been the mainstay of treatment until the advent of human insulin. Highly purified pork and beef preparations are still available and preferred by some. 'Human' insulin constitutes 80% of current production using recombinant DNA technology in genetically programmed yeast or bacteria. The advantage of this method is the ease of production of large quantities not reliant on animal sources, reduced immunogenicity and comparable efficacy. Several preparations with differing duration of action are available. The mode of treatment has improved with the introduction of discrete metered-dose and self-administered injection systems. Currently it is not possible to mimic the minute-to-minute and hour-to-hour variability of physiological insulin secretion. Current quick-acting insulins require at least 30 minutes before a meal is taken to allow dissociation of the hexameric form to the active monomeric form with subsequent absorption into the circulation. This is also influenced by variations in local circulation and fatty change at the injection site (lipodystrophy). Longer-acting versions aim to provide a background low-level concentration but suffer from the same bioavailability problems.

New insulin analogues have come into use that allow approximation to the physiological secretion of nondiabetics. The new analogues (so-called 'designer insulins' such as insulin lispro) have a similar action to insulin but have an altered amino-acid sequence. This is achieved by interchanging a lysine and proline at positions 28 and 29 in the human insulin beta chain that encourages the dissociated state. Thus, there is a rapid absorption of analogue into and loss from the circulation. This allows an injection immediately before eating to take effect in a similar way to that observed in normal subjects by reducing the postprandial glucose levels to near normal, with consequently less hypoglycaemia in the preprandial period. Conversely, there is a tendency, before the next meal, for preprandial levels of glucose to be raised. This is reflected in levels of glycosylated haemoglobin, which overall remain the same as those achieved with conventional insulin regimens. Only short-acting analogues are available at present and, until long-acting analogues become available, the problem of preprandial hyperglycaemia remains.

Treatment regimens for type 1 diabetes are wholly dependent on insulin. Those with type 2 diabetes who have poor control may also benefit from insulin. The long-term benefit of good control is a reduction in microvascular disease throughout the body but the disadvantage is an increase in the incidence of hypoglycaemia. Regimens should aim to provide sufficient basal activity between meals or times of metabolic stress to avoid hyperglycaemia and hypoglycaemia. Current basal-bolus regimens use combinations of intermediate-acting insulin twice daily and short-acting soluble insulin before meals, thus avoiding hypoglycaemia for much of the time. Future regimens could use a mixture of ultrashort-acting analogues and soluble insulin, thereby reducing postprandial glucose concentration and the incidence of hypoglycaemia. Where patients are achieving good control, there is no reason to change regimen.

The monitoring of diabetic care is a shared responsibility between patient and clinic. Current self-monitoring involves using blood glucose dipsticks and a finger-prick blood sample measured in a glucometer that has to be regularly calibrated. This gives an accurate and rapid level best performed before a meal. Glucometer values may not accurately correlate with serum levels but any changes are usually indicative of a change in insulin requirement. These levels are recorded in a diary and, combined with the patient's experience of their illness, can give them the cue to adjust their dose. Education of patients on the mechanism of their disease and anticipation of problems is crucial to the success of self-treatment for both short- and long-term control. This can be achieved by regular contact with diabetic nurse specialists working in outpatient clinics as open-access resources, which allow patients to monitor and self-treat with confidence. The general practitioner may offer practice-based diabetic clinics at which the diabetic diary is reviewed. Here, a routine assessment of blood pressure, serum glycosylated haemoglobin ($HBA_1c$), retinopathy, renal function and neuropathy are made. Annual retinoscopy is arranged with an ophthalmologist to monitor or treat retinopathy. At annual or biannual specialist clinic visits, further assessments are made. Where patients are having problems with hypoglycaemia, self-treatment with glucagon should be taught.

## Relevance to fertility

In mammals, reproductive function is highly sensitive to availability of food substrate. Although there is no direct evidence, it is likely that alterations in nutrition influence pulsatile release of GnRH in the forebrain, which may account for infertility in poorly controlled diabetes mellitus.

There is a general acceptance that type 1 diabetes predisposes to a higher incidence of first-trimester miscarriage, at one time estimated to be 26–30% overall, although this has reduced to 15.6% more recently, possibly due to an improvement in glycaemic control. In a prospective case–control study of 386 pregnant women with type 1 diabetes, 62 (16.1%) with diabetes and 70 (16.2%) controls had pregnancy losses within 21 days of conception. Of the women whose diabetes was well controlled, those who aborted had higher fasting and postprandial glucose levels in the first trimester than those who proceeded to deliver. In those with poorly controlled diabetes an increase by one standard deviation above the range for $HBA_1c$ was associated with an increase of 3.1% in pregnancy loss.[3] Explanations for the increased miscarriage rate include the effect of maternal metabolic factors and abnormalities of fetal metabolism before the seventh week of pregnancy. *In vitro* studies using mouse preimplantation embryos show a high correlation between the number of undeveloped embryos cultured in human diabetic serum and blood concentrations of serum glucose, ketones (acetoacetate) and $HBA_1c$. Disorders of prostaglandin synthesis in the yolk sac have also been postulated. There is also evidence of deficient insulin receptor binding in the placentas of women with diabetes aborting at midtrimester compared with those achieving full-term pregnancies, which suggests that tight glycaemic control throughout pregnancy may optimise insulin receptor function. There is evidence of a role for leptin, a 16-KD protein coded by the obesity gene in fetal weight gain during the third trimester (which may be a risk factor for stillbirth). It has been demonstrated that leptin mRNA and protein levels in placentas of diabetic pregnancies are increased three- to five-fold in association with raised cord insulin levels independent of maternal levels. Levels are also raised in cord blood in large-for-gestational-age infants compared with appropriate-for-gestational-age infants.

## Relevance to pregnancy

The planning of pregnancy in established diabetics is crucial to a successful outcome for mother and child. The maternal and fetal complications of diabetes in pregnancy are many. In turn, pregnancy has a profound effect on diabetic control. These influences include the medical complications of accelerated retinopathy, nephropathy, neuropathy, poor control, weight gain and increasing insulin requirements during pregnancy. Pregnancy-related problems include hypertension, macrosomia, polyhydramnios, infection, pre-eclampsia and intrapartum difficulties for the mother, such as shoulder dystocia and caesarean section. In a cohort study in north-west England, 462 diabetic pregnancies were monitored over five years.[4] There were 351 (76%) live births, a 17% miscarriage rate, a 2% risk of stillbirth (25/1000 live births compared with a population rate of 5/1000) and an infant mortality of 19.9/1000 compared with 6.8/1000 in the general population. Congenital abnormalities were raised, at 94.0/1000 compared with 6.8/1000 live births in the general population; these included cardiac and craniospinal abnormalities (sacral agenesis). Obstetric complications include ketoacidosis, shoulder dystocia and preterm labour. Neonatal complications include a higher rate of respiratory distress syndrome in term deliveries, hypomagnesaemia, hypocalcaemia and jaundice.

Prepregnancy counselling, education, good control and prompt treatment of complications form the basis for improved outcome of pregnancy. In addition to checking rubella status and giving advice on smoking and folic acid supplements, it should be reinforced that good diabetic control before conception is associated with a lower risk of congenital malformation. These occur in the neural tube, cardiac structures and spine (sacral agenesis) between the fifth and ninth weeks of gestation. A prepregnancy clinic also gives the opportunity for women with type 2 diabetes to change oral hypoglycaemic agents and for women with type 1 diabetes to review their current regimen and adjust it according to daily requirements.

Women with pre-existing retinopathy need to be advised that rapid progression may ensue if control is poor, but they can be reassured that nephropathy is unlikely to deteriorate. However, in established cases of nephropathy there is an increased risk of premature delivery. Women with diabetes have an increased risk of ischaemic heart disease and, if there is pre-existing hypertension, treatment with pregnancy-compatible preparations is necessary; those on atenolol (associated with intrauterine growth restriction) or angiotensin-converting enzyme inhibitors (associated with oligohydramnios) will have to change to more suitable preparations. Dietary advice is important throughout pregnancy as weight gain (more than 20% above ideal BMI) will influence insulin requirements and affect absorption, making control difficult, especially at term. The ideal environment for prepregnancy counselling is with those who are likely to be caring for the patient in pregnancy. These are the specialist diabetic nurse, midwife, dietician and the obstetrician and physician working in a joint clinic. Those who are most in need of this care and the least likely to prepare for pregnancy are the adolescent age group. Inevitably, women with diabetes must be aware of the commitment and attention that they must give to their disease and acknowledge the effect on work, social and family life.

## Management of diabetes in pregnancy

In established diabetes, the aim of management follows that of the nonpregnant population. The effects of variable insulin effectiveness and of hyperemesis (more common as a result of autonomic neuropathy) early in pregnancy make control difficult. These changes make ketoacidosis and the need for acute medical care more likely. The aim is to maintain preprandial blood glucose concentrations at less than 6 mmol/l. This should be monitored three times daily before meals and again before bed. Monthly serum HBA$_1$c levels reflect the overall control over the preceding four to six weeks, aiming for levels of 6% or less. Glycosylated plasma proteins (fructosamine) reflect the control of the previous two weeks as an alternative. Predicting the degree of adverse outcome in pregnancy by monitoring serum HBA1c levels has been assessed. In a follow-up study of 161 patients in the first trimester, values greater than 6.4% were significantly correlated with adverse fetal outcome.[5]

Dietary advice for pregnant women does not fundamentally change from that in the nonpregnant state. This is best given by a dietician working in the joint antenatal clinic aiming to reduce excess weight and maintain diabetic control. The use of unrefined complex carbohydrates should make up 50% of the total calories, and high-fibre-content food (30–50 g/day) allows energy to be sequestered at a steady rate, avoiding hyperglycaemia in the postprandial period.

Women with impaired glucose tolerance should have a preprandial glucose series performed, either in hospital or by a dedicated nurse specialist, to ascertain the need for insulin treatment. If levels are consistently over 6 mmol/l, this will be necessary more frequently. Often, dietary advice for women with gestational diabetes and those with impaired glucose tolerance will prolong the treatment-free period by reducing postprandial hyperglycaemia and fasting levels.

The regimens for treatment are similar to prepregnancy and, using a basal-bolus approach, fine tuning is allowed according to monitored levels. This approach, using soluble and preprandial short-acting insulin, is the most common regimen in UK practice. It is important to support patients in making changes in dosage, which may double during pregnancy. Women who are newly diagnosed and have some basal insulin secretion will require particular support and education in managing the changing needs of their condition. With the emphasis on keeping serum glucose levels down, the incidence of hypoglycaemia increases. Partners of women who experience frequent 'hypos' should also be able to administer glucagon and know who to call for advice. It is also important to reassure women that there is no evidence that short episodes of hypoglycaemia affect fetal wellbeing.

## Managing the complications of diabetes in pregnancy

Hypertension, retinopathy and neuropathy can deteriorate rapidly in pregnancy and require prompt treatment. Safe antihypertensive drugs include methyldopa, nifedipine and labetalol (which has the least effect on fetal renal function). The aim is to maintain a diastolic blood pressure below 90–95 mmHg. Ideally, complete ocular examinations should be performed every trimester and within three months postpartum, with colour fundus photography and laser treatment for retinopathy as necessary. In the nonpregnant state, renal screening for microalbuminuria is predictive for long-term renal disease. For obstetricians, it is difficult to differentiate between changes associated with pre-eclampsia and those attributed to renal disease alone. In the presence of normal creatinine clearance, moderate proteinuria can be tolerated. However, if levels rise, then the prognosis is poor and termination of pregnancy may have to be considered. Nephrotic syndrome with a low serum albumin and oedema in the presence of normal renal function may be managed with the judicious use of diuretics under the supervision of renal physicians. If fetal growth and maternal liver function, platelet and urate levels are within normal limits then pre-eclampsia is less likely.

## Managing the complications of pregnancy in women with diabetes

The challenge for control before and during pregnancy in improving outcomes is clear, as there is a five-fold increase in the stillbirth rate in units working outwith regional guidelines, a risk that would apply to a large proportion of women in the UK.[4] This cohort was also found to have a three-fold increase in infant mortality and a ten-fold increase in the prevalence of congenital malformations. At a pathophysiological level, this excess may be explained by pathological changes in placental circulation and the effect of glycosylation on placental transfer of substrate and oxygen. Fetal growth acceleration (macrosomia) occurs in as many as

20–30% of diabetic pregnancies, even where there is good control. The Pederson hypothesis proposes a mechanism in which maternal hyperglycaemia results in fetal hyperglycaemia and hyperinsulinaemia with enhanced growth.[6] In such cases, growth restriction may also result in association with fetal hyperglycaemia and acidaemia. Monitoring such pregnancies using ultrasound scanning of growth is conducted as for a normal pregnancy. The increased amniotic fluid resulting in polyhydramnios associated with diabetic pregnancies can be measured as part of a biophysical profile together with fetal breathing movements, which are also independently affected by the condition. The frequency of fetal monitoring is dictated by the presence of abnormal fetal morphology or poor maternal control. This may take the form of daily day-assessment monitoring or admission for control of diabetes, fetal monitoring and ultrasound scanning. The decision to deliver early must be balanced against the risks of prematurity, respiratory distress syndrome, failed vaginal delivery and stillbirth, a major risk should pregnancy be prolonged.

The timing and mode of delivery are decided taking into account maternal and fetal condition. Preterm labour will require corticosteroids for fetal lung maturity but may, however, lead to maternal hyperglycaemia and it is therefore best reserved for imminent delivery rather than prophylaxis. Macrosomia, as assessed by ultrasound, does not exclude a trial of vaginal delivery by induction at 37–38 weeks of gestation. In an uncomplicated pregnancy, spontaneous onset or induction of labour by 40 weeks of gestation is the aim. In each case, fine control of blood glucose levels using a sliding scale of intravenous short-acting insulin will be required. Once labour has started, management is conducted according to the local unit protocol. As labour is associated with a marked decline in insulin requirements to about one to two units per hour, a standard regimen would be an infusion of 10% dextrose (10 g/hour) with a separate pump infusion of insulin aiming for glucose levels of 7 mmol/l. On induction of labour, long-acting insulin preparations are stopped, while maintaining short-acting insulins with hourly monitoring of blood glucose levels. In all cases of planned vaginal delivery, the possibility of shoulder dystocia must be discussed with the patient and partner. After completion of the third stage, insulin requirements rapidly return to prepregnancy levels. Women with gestational diabetes and those with impaired glucose tolerance requiring insulin in pregnancy should stop insulin and then have monitoring to establish the level of treatment required. For women with type 2 diabetes, oral hypoglycaemic preparations can recommence; if blood glucose levels return to normal, then dietary advice will suffice. All such women should have a random glucose test performed in the postpartum period (6–12 weeks). The long-term risk of developing type 2 diabetes for this group is 36%, with impaired glucose tolerance in 25% at 24 years of follow-up.

## Type 2 diabetes, hyperinsulinaemia and insulin resistance

The relationship between type 2 diabetes, insulin resistance and hyperinsulinism is complex and may be associated with PCOS. Type 2 diabetes affects 2–3% of the population and is especially prevalent in the elderly population. The greatest change in prevalence is, however, in a younger age group associated with increasing obesity. In this group, hyperinsulinism initially develops as a result of insulin resistance with normal serum glucose levels. This progresses to a state of hyperinsulinism and hyperglycaemia, with increasing insulin resistance associated with obesity, dyslipidaemia and hypertension (syndrome X). The fundamental defect is thought to rest with insulin resistance. This has been attributed to a change in insulin-induced receptor phosphorylation and a post-insulin-binding defect in half of all cases associated with PCOS. PCOS features the symptoms of hyperandrogenism, menstrual dysfunction, weight gain and subfertility, with the signs of truncal redistribution of body fat and acanthosis nigricans in diabetics. In combination with the classic ultrasound finding of multiple peripheral ovarian cysts and dense ovarian stroma, these symptoms represent an extreme presentation of PCOS. The other extreme is represented by so-called 'lean' PCOS with the classic ultrasound features but a normal BMI and insulin resistance (see Chapters 8 and 9).

The aim of treatment of type 2 diabetes is to maintain strict normoglycaemia, as better control can lead to a reduction in major diabetic retinopathy by 25% and early nephropathy by 30%. Treatment centres on dietary control through education and the use of oral hypoglycaemic agents, although the results of the UK Prospective Diabetic Survey suggest that aggressive treatment, including insulin supplementation, may be necessary. The management of insulin resistance is the key goal. The traditional therapeutic options include the sulphonylureas, which augment insulin secretion (glibenclamide, gliclazide and tolbutamide), and the biguanides (e.g. metformin), which increase peripheral insulin sensitivity and decrease gluconeogenesis. A new class of agents, the proliferator-activated receptor-gamma agonists (thiazolidinediones or glitazones), such as rosiglitazone, act via nuclear receptors. These are peroxisome proliferator-activated receptors that modulate intracellular insulin sensitivity. There is a resultant improvement in glucose handling in fat, liver and skeletal muscle. There is evidence that free fatty acids are also reduced, leading to a direct reduction in endogenous insulin secretion. This preparation can be used with other agents to improve control without an increased risk of hypoglycaemia and without the anxiety of hepatotoxicity associated with its predecessor troglitazone.

In the context of subfertility featuring clomifene-resistant anovulation in women with PCOS who are not diabetic, co-treatment with metformin has shown subsequently to increase ovulation rates. This suggests that, in subclinical disease, correcting insulin resistance may have a role in correcting anovulation (see Chapter 9). Many of the long-term sequelae of PCOS also appear secondary to the development of impaired glucose tolerance and type 2 diabetes.

# References

1 World Health Organization. *Expert Committee on Diabetes Mellitus: Second Report.* Technical Report Series No. 646. Geneva: WHO; 1980.

2 Lind T. A prospective multicentre study to determine the influence of pregnancy upon the 75 g oral glucose tolerance test. In: Sutherland HW, Stowers JM, Person DWM, editors. *Carbohydrate Metabolism in Pregnancy and the Newborn IV.* Berlin: Springer; 1989. p. 209–26.

3 Mills JL, Simpson JL, Driscoll SG, Jovanovic-Peterson L, Van Allen M, Aarons JH, *et al.* Incidence of spontaneous abortion among normal women and insulin-dependent diabetic women whose pregnancies were identified within 21 days of conception. *N Engl J Med* 1988;**319**:1617–23.

4 Casson IF, Clarke CA, Howard CV, McKendrick O, Pennycook S, Pharoah PO, *et al.* Outcomes of pregnancy in insulin dependent diabetic women: results of a five year population cohort study. *BMJ* 1997;**315**:275–8.

5 Neilson GL, Sorenson HT, Neilson PH, Sabroe S, Olsen J. Glycosylated haemoglobin as predictor of adverse fetal outcome in type 1 diabetic pregnancies. *Acta Diabetol* 1997;**34**:217–22.

6 Pederson J. *The Pregnant Diabetic and her Newborn: Problems and Management.* Copenhagen: Munksgaard; 1977.

# 15 Lipid metabolism and lipoprotein transport

Fat absorbed from the diet and lipids synthesised by the liver and adipose tissue must be transported between the various tissues and organs for use and storage. As lipids are insoluble in water, the nonpolar lipids (triglycerides and cholesterol esters) are associated with amphipathic lipids (phospholipids and cholesterol) and proteins to make water-miscible lipoproteins. Lipids are transported in plasma as lipoproteins. Pure fat is less dense than water; therefore, as the proportion of lipid to protein in a lipoprotein increases, the density decreases. In addition to free fatty acids, there are four major groups of lipoproteins. These are:

- chylomicrons, derived from intestinal absorption of triacylglycerol
- very-low-density lipoproteins (VLDL), derived from the liver for the export of triacylglycerides
- low-density lipoproteins (LDL), representing a final stage in the catabolism of VLDL
- high-density lipoprotein (HDL) involved in VLDL and cholesterol metabolism and also in cholesterol transport.

Triacylglycerol is the predominant lipid in chylomicrons and VLDL (larger complexes), while cholesterol and phospholid are the predominant lipids in LDL and HDL (smaller complexes). A typical lipoprotein consists of a lipid core of mainly nonpolar triglyceride and cholesterol ester surrounded by a single surface layer of amphipathic phospholipid and free cholesterol and protein molecules. The protein moiety is known as apolipoprotein, constituting as much as 60% of HDL or as little as 1% of chylomicron particles. Some apolipoproteins are integral and cannot be removed, while others are free to transfer to other lipoproteins.

One or more apolipoproteins are present in each lipoprotein. The major apolipoprotein in HDL is apoA; that in LDL is apoB, which is also present in VLDL and chylomicrons. The other apolipoproteins include the apoC group, which are smaller polypeptides that are freely transferable between several lipoproteins. The free fatty acids (nonesterified fatty acids, unesterified fatty acids) arise in plasma from lipolysis of triglycerides in adipose tissue or as a result of the action of lipoprotein lipase during uptake of triglycerides in tissue. They are found in combination with albumin, which is highly effective at achieving solubility. Low levels of fatty acids are recorded in the fully fed state, rising in the post-absorptive phase and peaking in the fully fasted state. The rate of removal of free fatty acids from the blood is extremely rapid, some of the uptake being used for an oxidative state, and free fatty acids supply 25–50% of the energy requirements during fasting. In a fasting state, the cholesterol measured is that of LDL and serum triglycerides are a measure of VLDL. Cholesterol in HDL and LDL can be separated and quantified by simple precipitation methods.

The plasma lipoproteins are interrelated components and together are responsible for the complex process of lipid transport and homeostasis. There are two main sources of lipid in the plasma: dietary fat and hepatic synthesis.

## Transport of dietary fat

The average Western daily diet contains approximately 120 g of fat and 0.5–1.0 g of cholesterol. Almost all of the glyceride and about half of the cholesterol is assimilated and re-esterified in the intestinal cells and packaged to form large chylomicron particles. When the particles enter the lacteals of the intestinal mesentery they contain two main apolipoproteins, A1 and B. Following its transit through the thoracic duct into plasma it acquires apolipoproteins C and E primarily by transfer from HDL. ApoCIII activates the enzyme lipoprotein lipase in the endothelial cells of the capillary bed of adipose tissue and striated muscles and then causes lipolysis of the chylomicron particles to release glycerol and fatty acids. This process also releases the phospholipid and protein surface coat into the HDL pool. The delipidation process leaves the chylomicron remnant, which undergoes conformational changes and is taken up by hepatocytes delivering dietary cholesterol to the liver (Figure 15.1).

Chylomicrons transport dietary lipids via lymph into plasma and then are degraded to cholesterol remnants by extrahepatic lipoprotein lipase, which is activated by apoCII. Chylomicron remnants are taken up by the hepatic receptors, which recognise the apoE on their surface. This forms one source of cholesterol for the liver. VLDL carry endogenously synthesised triglycerides from the liver into plasma, where, like chylomicrons, they undergo lipolysis by the enzyme lipoprotein lipase, undergoing partial degradation to form VLDL remnants or intermediate-density lipoprotein (IDL). These are then either taken up by LDL receptors, which recognise the apoE and apoB that they contain, or further degraded to form LDL particles that contain apoB but no apoE. Hepatic lipase may be involved in

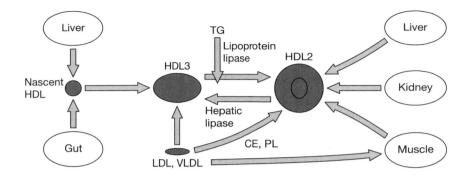

**Figure 15.1** Cholesterol transport by high-density cholesterol (HDL); CE, cholesterol ester; LDL, low-density cholesterol; PL, phospholipid; TG, triglycerides

this process. LDL then undergoes catabolism via at least two major pathways, one of which is mediated by the LDL receptor.

HDL is of diverse origin, its lipids being derived from free cholesterol and phospholipids released during the lipolysis of chylomicrons and VLDL, as well as free cholesterol effluxing from peripheral cells. An HDL cycle has been proposed to account for the transfer of cholesterol from tissues to the liver, a process called reverse cholesterol transport. This process involves uptake of and esterification of cholesterol by HDL$_3$ by the enzyme lecithin cholesterol acyltransferase, which becomes less dense, forming HDL$_2$. Hepatic lipase hydrolyses HDL phospholipid and triglycerides, allowing the particle to release its cargo of cholesterol esters to the liver, whereupon the particle becomes more dense, reforming HDL$_3$, which re-enters the cycle.

## HEPATIC LIPID METABOLISM

Most lipid pathways converge or originate in the liver, making the liver central to the maintenance of lipid homeostasis and prevention of atherosclerosis. Hepatic cholesterol may be derived from dietary sources or from endogenous synthesis. The cholesterol may be stored as cytoplasmic ester droplets, secreted in bile, converted to bile acids or exported in lipoproteins. Most of the plasma VLDL is of hepatic origin. VLDLs are vehicles of transport for triglycerides from the liver to extrahepatic sites and share the metabolic pathway of chylomicrons with a similar protein component as apolipoprotein B. VLDL has the same delipidation pathway and has a similar exchange of components to HDL. ApoB of hepatic origin is of greater molecular weight than that produced

compared with an equal number of women who were still menstruating. The results were adjusted for age of both groups. There was an increase in plasma LDL cholesterol, with reduction in HDL cholesterol. Jensen *et al.*[2] performed another prospective study that showed elevated total cholesterol, triglycerides and LDL cholesterol concentrations. The decrease in HDL cholesterol was not marked, although there was a redistribution of cholesterol within the HDL spectrum. A third cross-sectional study by Stevenson *et al.*[3] confirmed the above findings, including decreased levels of HDL cholesterol, as well as $HDL_2$ and $HDL_3$ cholesterol in post-menopausal women. The menopause affects all subtypes of LDL cholesterol, particularly lipoprotein(a), which is reported to increase by 50% after the menopause, thereby increasing risk of coronary heart disease.

Bilateral oophorectomy provides a useful model for the effect of the menopause on lipoproteins without the confounding effect of age. Increase in triglycerides and total and LDL cholesterol have been reported that are consistent with the withdrawal of estrogen. However, there is no evidence that HDL cholesterol levels are adversely affected, although subtle changes in composition cannot be excluded. The apparent premenopausal protection afforded by estrogen is thought to be mediated by the suppression of hepatic lipase activity by estrogen with elevated levels of HDL cholesterol and decreased levels of LDL cholesterol.

To summarise, loss of ovarian function appears to adversely affect the lipid profile by increasing levels of triglycerides and total and LDL cholesterol. The evidence that HDL cholesterol levels contribute to this risk has not been consistent. This is similar to the report that HDL cholesterol is not affected by female puberty or the menstrual cycle.

Estrogen replacement therapy has a beneficial effect on the lipid profile by lowering plasma LDL cholesterol and elevating HDL cholesterol. However, oral estrogen may increase the levels of plasma triglycerides, an effect that may not be evident with other routes of administration.

## References

1 Matthews KA, Meilahn E, Kuller LH, Kelsey LF, Cagguila AW, Wing RR. Menopause and risk factors for coronary heart disease. *N Engl J Med* 1989;**321**:641–6.

2 Jensen J, Nilas L, Christiansen C. Influence of menopause on serum lipids and lipoproteins. *Maturitas* 1990;**12**:321–31.

3 Stevenson JC, Crook D, Godsland IF. Influence of age and menopause on serum lipids and lipoproteins in healthy women. *Atherosclerosis* 1993;**98**:83–90.

# 16 Premature ovarian failure

Premature ovarian failure is defined as the cessation of ovarian function under the age of 40 years and occurs in approximately 1% of women. In order to have an understanding of the aetiology of ovarian failure, which is still unknown in many cases, it is important first to have an idea of the factors that influence ovarian ageing.

## The control of ovarian ageing

The control of ovarian ageing is still one of the greatest enigmas in reproductive biology. The function of the ovary depends upon the total number of oocytes contained within primordial follicles. Primordial follicles and oocytes are derived during fetal life and the oogonial stem cell line is lost before birth (see Chapter 1). The final number of oocytes is determined by three factors:

- the maximum number achieved by mitotic divisions
- the time at which they enter meiosis, preventing further increase in number
- the rate of atresia.

The factors that affect the number of mitotic divisions and the transition from mitosis to meiosis are unknown.

More germs cells die during fetal life than survive in primordial follicles. The maximum number of germs cells is approximately seven million and this is achieved at 20 weeks of gestation. By birth, this is reduced to between one and two million. It is thought that the eliminated germ cells might have a higher rate of chromosomal abnormalities than those that remain, although this has never been conclusively proven.

The number of primordial follicles at puberty has been mathematically related to the final adult weight of a particular species and the lifespan of a species is also related to the number of primordial follicles at puberty. In all species, the primordial follicle number declines with age. The size of the follicle store is not directly related to the rate of ovulation but is related to the daily fraction recruited, which changes with age. Recruitment of primordial follicles occurs throughout life and is initially independent of

FSH. Indeed, the FSH receptor is expressed only at the primary follicle stage. The growing fraction of primordial follicles appears to be upregulated when the total numbers are reduced, and this explains the increased rate of loss in humans with age.[1] The accelerated rate of depletion in older ovaries is due more to the initiation of growth than atresia, although the control mechanisms are still to be elucidated. From birth to puberty, approximately 75% of the follicle store is lost. At puberty about 250 000 follicles remain and, between puberty and menopause, there is the potential for up to about 500 ovulations.

Menopause occurs when there are approximately 1000 follicles left in the ovary. Postmenopausally, therefore, some follicles do remain but they do not grow to maturity, perhaps because high circulating levels of FSH cause receptor downregulation. A number of mathematical models have been developed to express the rate of decline of primordial follicle number.[2] When 10 000 follicles remain the menopause will occur in approximately 5–10 years, and when there are 100 000 remaining menopause will be in 21.5–26.5 years. At the age of 25 years, approx-imately 37 follicles leave the human ovary by either growth or atresia daily (in other words, approximately 1000 per month), while at the age of 45 years this falls to approximately two per day. The rate of ovarian ageing appears to be intrinsically determined and the half-life of the follicle population is approximately seven years, increasing exponentially with a doubling of the exponential rate after the age of about 37.5 years (Figure 16.1).

If the rate of follicle loss did not increase, then the menopause could be expected to occur at approximately 71 years of age. The reason for the menopause occurring is unclear and it may actually represent an extension of life due to increased nutrition and wellbeing of the human population rather than a physiological feature in itself. With respect to the recruitment of the primordial follicles, this is due to unknown processes in cellular metabolism and signalling and no physiological interventions are able to halt recruitment. Thus, recruitment occurs while an individual is pregnant and also while she is taking the contraceptive pill.

The frequency distribution of the age at menopause has been described by Treloar[3] in 763 American women. The age of menopause appears to be similar in all Western communities, although women in developing countries appear to have a menopause five or six years earlier and this may be a reflection of undernutrition during fetal life, as nutritional status during infant or adult life does not appear to have a direct bearing on ovarian ageing.

Using mathematical models for the ageing of the ovary, devised from data of follicle counts at different ages together with projected mean ages at menopause, Faddy et al.[4] have developed certain algorithms. For example, it has been suggested that the surgical loss of one ovary is not

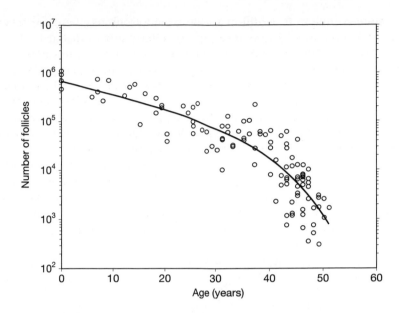

**Figure 16.1** Decline in oocytes with age (Faddy and Gosden[2])

likely to hasten the menopause by more than seven years – in other words, beyond the age of 44 years, by which time 5% of the population are menopausal. If 50% of the follicle store is lost by the age of 30 years, then the expected age of menopause is 44 years; for each further year that a 50% reduction has occurred, the menopause will be delayed by 0.6 years. Thus, if 50% have been lost by the age of 37.5 years, the menopause can be expected to occur at the age of 48 years. On the other hand, if 90% of the follicle store is lost by the age of 14 years, another 13 years of ovarian activity can be expected, with a menopause occurring at the age of 27 years; for each further year that a 90% reduction has occurred, the menopause will be delayed by 0.6 years, so that if 90% have been lost at the age of 37.5 years the menopause will occur at the age of 41 years (Figure 16.1).

Atresia and apoptosis (programmed physiological cell death) are initiated by genes that code for effector proteins (which lead to cell death in response to external stimuli) and occur once the follicle has passed its primary stage. Follicles that are not selected for ovulation undergo atresia at the later preantral or early antral stage (1–5 mm in diameter), when continued growth would be FSH-dependent. Follicles destined for atresia can be rescued by FSH administration and the oocyte remains healthy until late stages of atresia, at which point it will resume meiosis due to loss of the cumulous complex. In addition to the gonadotrophins, there are several hormonal inhibitors of apoptosis, whose effects are mediated by IGF-1, transforming growth factor-α, keratinocyte growth factor, hepatocyte growth factor, estradiol, progesterone, vasoactive intestinal peptide and protein kinase activators. It is also important that extracellular matrix interaction and gap junctions are appropriately maintained. There are several intracellular effectors of ovarian cell death, for example *bcl-2*, which is a proto-oncogene, *bcl-x long* and *bax*. Interleukin-converting enzyme and its analogues and p53 are also inducers of apoptosis, as are a number of other messengers. There are various repressors of apoptosis, including BCL-2, BCL-X long, superoxide dismutase and glutathione peroxidase. Initiators and repressors of apoptosis are constantly being evaluated but it appears that it is not the induction of apoptosis itself that effects ovarian ageing but rather the recruitment of the primordial follicles to growth.

## Definition and diagnosis

Premature ovarian failure is the cessation of periods accompanied by raised gonadotrophin concentrations before the age of 40 years. It can occur at any age. The exact incidence of this condition is unknown, as many cases go unrecognised, but estimates are 1–5% of the female population.[5] In a study of 1858 women, the incidence was 1 in 1000 by the age of 30 years and 1 in 100 by the age of 40 years.[5] Studies of amenorrhoeic women report the incidence of premature ovarian failure to be between 10% and 36%.

Before the absolute cessation of periods of true premature ovarian failure, some women experience an intermittent return to menses, interspersed between variable periods of amenorrhoea. Gonadotrophin levels usually remain moderately elevated during these spontaneous cycles, with plasma FSH concentrations of 15–20 iu/l. This occult or incipient ovarian failure, or 'resistant ovary syndrome', is associated with the presence of primordial follicles on ovarian biopsy. Ovarian biopsy is no longer recommended in the assessment of these cases because a single sample is not reliably representative and will not help with management. Occasionally, pregnancies occur spontaneously in patients with resistant ovary syndrome. Ovulation induction is of no benefit, as the ovaries are usually as resistant to exogenous gonadotrophins as they are to endogenous hormones. It is probable that reports of pregnancy in women with premature ovarian failure represent cases of fluctuating ovarian function rather than successes of treatment.

Measurements of serum concentrations of FSH, estradiol and inhibin have been used to assess 'ovarian reserve', as have various ovarian stimulation or 'challenge' tests and ultrasound scans of ovarian volume, blood flow and antral follicle number. None of these tests, however, has been shown to indicate how many more ovulations a woman may have or when they will occur. Thus, if a woman with resistant ovary syndrome or incipient ovarian failure and symptoms of estrogen deficiency wishes to conceive, she should be advised to take an HRT preparation, which will not inhibit ovulation (or adversely affect a pregnancy). On the other hand, if a pregnancy would be unwanted, it is important to advise the use of either an oral contraceptive preparation or contraception together with HRT.

If a woman has amenorrhoea and an elevated serum FSH concentration (greater than 20 iu/l) on more than two occasions, it is likely that she has premature ovarian failure. The longer the period of amenorrhoea and the higher the FSH level, the greater the likelihood that the ovarian failure is permanent. A single elevated FSH level, even if greater than 40 iu/l, should be treated with caution, as spontaneous ovulation and pregnancy have still been observed. Once the diagnosis of premature ovarian failure has been made, further specific endocrinological tests are unnecessary. Additional investigations include karyotyping, screening for auto-antibodies and associated autoimmune disease if relevant and a baseline assessment of bone mineral density. As always, a detailed history is important, with particular attention to a family history of premature ovarian failure, autoimmune disease. The possibility of ovarian failure secondary to infections (including mumps and HIV) should be considered.

## Causation

In approximately two-thirds of cases, the cause of ovarian failure cannot be identified.[6] It is unknown whether these cases are truly 'idiopathic' or due to as yet undiscovered genetic, immunological or environmental factors. A series of 323 women with premature ovarian failure attending an endocrinology clinic in London identified 23% with Turner syndrome, 6% after chemotherapy, 4% with familial premature ovarian failure and 2% each who had pelvic surgery, pelvic irradiation, galactosaemia and 46,XY gonadal dysgenesis.[6] Viral and bacterial infection may also lead to ovarian failure – thus, infections such as mumps and cytomegalovirus or HIV in adult life can adversely affect long-term ovarian function, as can severe pelvic inflammatory disease. Ovarian failure before puberty is usually due to a chromosomal abnormality or a childhood malignancy that required chemotherapy or radiotherapy – from which, parenthetically, there are increasing numbers of survivors into adulthood with premature ovarian failure. The likelihood of developing ovarian failure after therapy for cancer is difficult to predict but the age of the patient is a significant factor – the younger the patient, the greater the follicle pool and the better her chances of retaining ovarian function. Environmental toxins might be a factor in causing premature ovarian failure and this is an area of continuing research. The best-known toxin is cigarette smoke, which has been shown to lower the age of menopause.

## GENETIC CAUSES

Chromosomal abnormalities are relatively common in women with premature ovarian failure. Adolescents who lose ovarian function soon after menarche are often found to have a Turner mosaic (46,XX/45,X) or an X-chromosome trisomy (47,XXX). There are many genes on the X chromosome that are essential for normal ovarian function. It would appear that two active X chromosomes are required during fetal life in order to lay down a normal follicle store. In fetuses with Turner syndrome, normal numbers of oocytes appear on the genital ridge but accelerated atresia takes place during late fetal life. Thus, streak gonads occur and it is only the mosaic form of Turner syndrome that permits any possibility of ovarian function. X mosaicisms are the most common chromosomal abnormality in reported series of premature ovarian failure, ranging from 5% to 40%.[7] Other X-chromosome anomalies may result in ovarian failure, for example balanced translocations in the long arm of chromosome X between Xq13 and Xq26, which is a critical region for ovarian function.

### Turner syndrome

Turner syndrome is the most common cause of gonadal dysgenesis. In its most severe form, the 45,X genotype is associated with the classical Turner features, including short stature, webbing of the neck, cubitus valgus, widely spaced nipples, cardiac and renal abnormalities and, often, autoimmune hypothyroidism. Spontaneous menstruation may occur, particularly when there is mosaicism, but premature ovarian failure usually ensues. It is important to determine the karyotype because the presence of a Y chromosome in an individual with gonadal dysgenesis necessitates removal of gonadal tissue because of an increased risk of malignancy. Serum gonadotrophin concentrations are elevated compared with adolescents of the same age and may approach the menopausal range.

Management includes low-dose estrogen therapy to promote breast development without further disturbing linear growth; treatment with growth hormone has also benefited some individuals. Cyclical estrogen plus progestogen may be used as maintenance therapy. Spontaneous conception has been reported in patients with Turner syndrome, but this is rare. However, the possibility of assisted conception and oocyte donation should be discussed at an early age.

# Fragile X syndrome

The fragile X syndrome is the most common inherited cause of learning disability, with a prevalence of 1:4000 in males and 1 in 8000 in females. It is characterised by a heterogeneous mixture of physical, behavioural and cognitive features. Most published information refers to fragile X syndrome in males, of whom about 80% are moderately to severely mentally restricted, while females usually display a milder phenotype, with a borderline IQ of 70–85. Fragile X syndrome is an X-linked dominant disorder with reduced penetration. Unaffected carriers in a family have an increased risk of transmitting the disorder to successive generations. Changes in the DNA sequence appear to occur during oogonial mitotic divisions. The disorder is due to a mutation in a gene on the long arm of the X chromosome, which includes a trinucleotide repeat sequence (CGG) in the 5' untranslated region (FRAXA site) of the first of its 17 exons. The gene is known as *'fragile X mental restriction-1'* (*FMR-1*, Xq27.3), which transcribes a cytoplasmic protein that is found in all cells but in a higher concentration in the ovary, brain and testis. It is the absence of this protein that results in the fragile X syndrome phenotype. In normal individuals, there are fewer than 50 trinucleotide repeats; those with a premutation have between 50 and 200 trinucleotide repeats and those with the full mutation in excess of 200.

Affected families have mutations in the *FMR-1* gene, leading to hereditary instability. These mutations can be of variable sizes, the largest resulting in a 'full mutation', while smaller mutations are known as 'premutations'. As somatic cells in females have a randomly inactivated X chromosome, only half of females with the full mutation have a fragile X phenotype. Women with a premutation are phenotypically normal but appear to have a significantly increased risk of premature ovarian failure. The largest series of 395 premutation carriers found 16.0% with premature ovarian failure compared with 0.4% of a control population.[8] When looking specifically at series of women with premature ovarian failure, the premutation carrier status is 4.0–6.0%, compared with 0.4% in the normal population. It is interesting that women with the full mutation appear to have a normal ovarian lifespan and the reason for the premutation leading to premature ovarian failure is at present unknown. The implications are of importance not only for the females in a family of carriers but also, of course, for their offspring.

## FAMILIAL FACTORS

There are several syndromes that are associated with premature ovarian failure, such as familial blepharophimosis, in which the abnormality is on chromosome 3. Galactosaemia is another rare example, in which a metabolic defect has a direct inhibitory effect on ovarian function, probably due to a build-up of galactose within the ovary that decreases the initial number of oogonia.

There is evidence for strong genetic factors determining the age of the menopause. Interest has recently turned to specific familial forms of premature ovarian failure in which abnormalities are present in the critical region of the long arm of the X chromosome from Xq13 to Xq26. At least two genetic variants have been identified, the *POF-1* gene (Xq21.3–q27) and the *POF-2* gene (Xq13.3–q21.1). The latter appears to be of paternal origin and leads to a lower age of onset of ovarian failure than those who have *POF-1* deletions. Epidemiological studies have suggested a familial premature ovarian failure rate of approximately 30%. A series of 71 women with premature ovarian failure revealed a familial incidence of 31% and there was a significantly higher age of menopause in those with familial failure compared with those with sporadic failure (37.5 versus 31.0 years).[9]

## AUTOIMMUNE CAUSES

Ovarian autoantibodies can be measured and have been found in up to 69% of cases of premature ovarian failure. However, the assays are expensive and not readily available in most units. It is therefore important to consider other autoimmune disorders and screen for autoantibodies to the thyroid gland, gastric mucosa parietal cells and adrenal gland if there is any clinical indication. There are several potential ovarian antigens and the potential for autoantibody formation has been long recognised. The clinical significance of antiovarian antibodies is uncertain, particularly as their concentrations fluctuate and do not always relate to the severity of disease. It is therefore uncertain whether antiovarian antibodies are pathogenic or secondary to antigen-release after ovarian damage. Some researchers have, however, failed to identify receptor autoantibodies in patients with premature ovarian failure and debate in this area continues.[7]

# Management

The diagnosis and consequences of premature ovarian failure require careful counselling of the patient. It may be particularly difficult for a young woman to accept the need for taking estrogen preparations that are clearly labelled as being intended for older postmenopausal women, while at the same time having to come to terms with the inability to conceive naturally. The short- and long-term consequences of ovarian failure and estrogen deficiency are similar to those occurring in the fifth and sixth decade. However, the duration of the problem is much longer and therefore HRT is advisable to reduce the consequences of estrogen deficiency in the long term.

Younger women with premature loss of ovarian function have an increased risk of osteoporosis. A study of 200 amenorrhoeic women between the ages of 16 and 40 years demonstrated a mean reduction in bone mineral density of 15%, as compared with a control group and after correction for body weight, smoking and exercise.[10] The degree of bone loss was correlated with the duration of the amenorrhoea and the severity of the estrogen deficiency rather than the underlying diagnosis, and was worse in patients with primary amenorrhoea than in those with secondary amenorrhoea. A return to normal estrogen status may improve bone mass density, but bone mineral density is unlikely to improve by more than 5–10% and it probably does not return to its normal value. However, it is not certain whether the radiological improvement seen will actually reduce the risk of fracture, as remineralisation is not equivalent to restrengthening of bone. Early diagnosis and early correction of estrogen status are therefore important.

Women with premature ovarian failure have an increased risk of cardiovascular disease. Estrogens have been shown to have beneficial effects on cardiovascular status in women. They increase the levels of cardioprotective high-density lipoprotein but also total triglyceride levels, while decreasing total cholesterol and low-density lipoprotein levels. The overall effect is of cardiovascular protection.

Women with hypoestrogenic amenorrhoea require hormone replacement. A cyclical estrogen/progestogen preparation is required for patients with a uterus in order to prevent endometrial hyperplasia, which is a high-risk consequence of prolonged unopposed estrogen therapy. The HRT preparations prescribed for menopausal women are also preferred for young women. The reason for this is that even modern low-dose combined oral contraceptive preparations contain at least twice the amount of estrogen that is recommended for HRT, in order to achieve a contraceptive suppressive effect on the hypothalamic-pituitary axis. HRT also contains 'natural' estrogens rather than the synthetic ethinyl-estradiol that is found in most oral contraceptives.

It should be noted that there is mounting evidence to suggest a slight increase in the risk of developing breast cancer with longer durations of HRT therapy. However, it is difficult to extrapolate these large studies to small numbers of younger women, who constitute a separate population with different risk factors. On balance, the beneficial effects of hormone replacement in reducing osteoporosis and cardiovascular mortality are thought to outweigh the risk of breast cancer, particularly in women with premature ovarian failure. Although HRT is likely to be advantageous to the future wellbeing of a woman with premature ovarian failure, it is also important to advise on general measures to minimise the detrimental effects of amenorrhoea that may have occurred before the problem was recognised. It is therefore important to advise against cigarette smoking and to advocate a balanced diet, exercise and maintenance of a normal BMI.

Follow-up of women with premature ovarian failure should be at least on an annual basis to monitor HRT, detect the development of associated diseases and provide appropriate support and counselling.

## OOCYTE DONATION

Oocyte donation can be used to treat women with premature ovarian failure, of whatever cause. Extensive counselling is required of both partners and the donor, who might be undergoing assisted conception herself or have an altruistic desire to donate eggs and thereby undergo an IVF cycle. Donor anonymity is preferred and leads to fewer long-term problems. The donor should be under the age of 36 years in order to reduce the chance of age-related chromosomal problems. This is the recommendation of the Human Fertilisation and Embryology Authority, which licenses assisted conception clinics in the UK.

It is necessary to provide the recipient with an artificial hormone replacement regimen, usually with increasing doses of oral estrogens, with the addition of natural progesterone three days before embryo transfer. Recipients who still have a spontaneous menstrual cycle require pituitary desensitisation before starting the hormone regimen, while amenorrhoeic women with ovarian failure do not. Interestingly, it is the latter group who appear to have better results, possibly because the HRT regimen has not been imposed on a pre-existing cycle. Close synchrony is required between the recipient's cycle and the donor's IVF cycle if fresh embryos (which provide better pregnancy rates than cryopreserved embryos) are to be transferred. The recipient is monitored using ultrasound measurements of endometrial thickness.

Pregnancy rates of about 30% per treatment cycle can be expected. The chance of conception declines with increasing age of the donor but also, less markedly, with increasing age of the recipient, presumably due to endometrial aging. The endometrial effect on implantation rates with oocyte donation is also apparent when the aetiology of the ovarian failure is examined, as the best pregnancy rates are achieved in women with premature ovarian failure who have an anatomically normal uterus. Women with Turner syndrome who have not undergone a spontaneous puberty and women who have received radiotherapy to the pelvis have reduced uterine blood flow and suboptimal endometrial development in response to exogenous estrogen therapy (sometimes radiotherapy destroys any subsequent endometrial function). These patients therefore do less well when undergoing oocyte donation. Furthermore, it would seem inadvisable to use the oocytes donated by a sister of a woman with premature ovarian failure, as they also appear to do less well than those of anonymous fertile donors.

## CRYOPRESERVATION OF OVARIAN TISSUE

Experimental work in animals has succeeded in transplanting primordial follicles into irradiated ovaries, with subsequent ovulation and normal pregnancy. An extension of this work has resulted in successful cryopreservation of human ovarian tissue[11,12] and reimplantation of the thawed tissue with resultant follicular growth, after stimulation with exogenous FSH. *In vitro* maturation of follicles from cryopreserved ovarian tissue is another possible method for obtaining mature oocytes for subsequent IVF. These techniques are still at an experimental stage and are undergoing further evaluation. The methods employed were devised for the preservation of fertility and ovarian function in young women before sterilising chemotherapy or radiotherapy. The potential exists for the cryopreservation of ovarian tissue for women destined to undergo ovarian failure: an event that might be predictable from genetic or family studies. Whether the cryopreserved ovarian tissue is genetically competent would, of course, be uncertain, but it is easy to foresee the day when women with fragile X permutations or Turner mosaicism might be asking for ovarian cryopreservation during their adolescent years. At the present time, however, appropriate advice would be for these women to aim for pregnancy using healthy donated oocytes.

# References

1 Gougeon A, Ecochard R, Thalabard JC. Age-related changes of the population of human ovarian follicles: increase in the disappearance rate of non-growing and early-growing follicles in aging women. *Biol Reprod* 1994;**50**:653–63.

2 Faddy MJ, Gosden RG. A model conforming the decline in follicle numbers to the age of menopause in women. *Hum Reprod* 1996;**11**:1484–6.

3 Treloar AE. Menstrual cyclicity and the pre-menopause. *Maturitas* 1981;**3**:249–64.

4 Faddy MJ, Gosden RG, Gougeon A, Richardson SJ, Nelson JF. Accelerated disappearance of ovarian follicles in mid-life: implications for forecasting menopause. *Hum Reprod* 1992;**7**:1342–6.

5 Coulam CB, Adamson SC, Annegers JF. Incidence of premature ovarian failure. *Obstet Gynecol* 1986;**67**:604–6.

6 Conway GS, Kaltas G, Patel A, Davies MC, Jacobs HS. Characterization of idiopathic premature ovarian failure. *Fertil Steril* 1996;**65**:337–41.

7 Anasti JN. Premature ovarian failure: an update. *Fertil Steril* 1998;**70**:1–15.

8 Allington-Hawkins DJ, Babul-Hirji R, Chitayat D, Holden JJ, Yang KT, Lee C, *et al.* Fragile X premutation is a significant risk factor for premature ovarian failure: the International Collaborative POF and Fragile X study – preliminary data. *Am J Med Genet* 1999;**83**:322–5.

9  Vegetti W, Grazia Tibiletti M, Testa G, de Lauretis Yankowski, Alagna F, Castoldi E, *et al*. Inheritance in idiopathic premature ovarian failure: analysis of 71 cases. *Hum Reprod* 1998;**13**:1796–800.

10 Davies MC, Hall ML, Jacobs HS. Bone mineral loss in young women with amenorrhoea. *BMJ* 1990;**301**:790–93.

11 Newton H, Aubard Y, Rutherford A, Sharma V, Gosden RG. Low temperature storage and grafting of human ovarian tissue. *Hum Reprod* 1996;**11**:1487–91.

12 Jadoul P, Donnez J, Dolmans MM, Squifflet J, Lengele B, Martinez-Madrid B. Laparoscopic ovariectomy for whole human ovary cryopreservation: technical aspects. *Fertil Steril* 2006; Dec 13 [Epub ahead of print].

# 17 Calcium metabolism and its disorders

Calcium plays an essential role in homeostasis. Serum levels of calcium are precisely controlled, principally through the actions of parathyroid hormone. Serum calcium is in a dynamic equilibrium with that bound to plasma albumin and that in bone as hydroxyapatite. The main sources of calcium in the diet are milk, cheese, leaf and, in particular, root vegetables, nuts, greens and 'hard' water. Absorption from dietary sources is inefficient, compounded by up to 1 g faecal loss and up to 500 mg urinary loss daily. Calcium absorption is reduced by oxalates in leaf vegetables and phytates in wholemeal flours and is increased by aciduric meat-derived protein, while urinary secretion is enhanced by high dietary sodium and reduced by potassium. The biochemistry of phosphorous is intimately involved with that of calcium. It is lost from the renal tract in exchange for calcium recovery under the influence of parathyroid hormone. The daily turnover of calcium is 25 mmol (25 mmol ingested in the diet, 20 mmol lost in the gut and 5 mmol lost in the urine). The turnover in bone calcium alone is 10 mmol per day from a total bone content of 25 mol (nearly 1300 g). In large part, the turnover of phosphorus mirrors that of calcium, with the larger proportion being lost from the kidney (40 mmol ingested, 15 mmol lost in faeces and 25 mmol lost in urine).

## Calcium and bone homeostasis

As 99% of total body calcium is contained within the skeletal system, the maintenance and control of calcium metabolism is vital. Bone as a material represents a dynamic, metabolically active, regenerative composite tissue. The cellular components of bone are chiefly osteoblasts, osteoclasts, progenitor cells and osteocytes. Osteoblasts are responsible for bone matrix formation (type 1 collagen and mucopolysaccharide), which subsequently become mineralised. Other products include collagenase, prostaglandin $E_2$ ($PGE_2$), bone-associated proteins, osteocalcin (a bone-specific marker in serum) and osteonectin. Osteocalcin, activated by vitamin K gamma-carboxylation, increases with new bone formation. Osteoblasts also have receptors for parathyroid hormone (PTH), calcitonin, calcitriol, $PGE_2$,

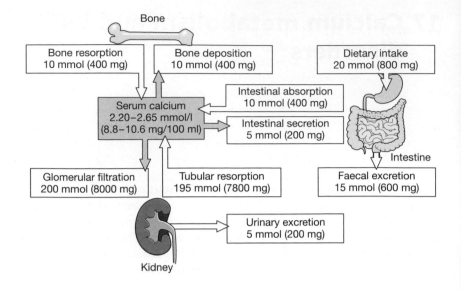

**Figure 17.1** Calcium homeostasis

corticosteroids, Interleukins 1α and 6 (IL-1α and IL-6) and various cytokines, e.g. transforming growth factors (TGF-β).[1] Osteoclasts are multinucleate cells that resorb calcified bone or cartilage and respond to PTH, PGE$_2$ and vitamin D via osteoblasts using an as yet undefined second-messenger system. Tumour necrosis factor activates osteoclastic activity associated with tumours (Figure 17.1).

The principal hormones involved in calcium homeostasis are PTH and calcitonin. PTH is synthesised by the parathyroid glands by sequential cleavage of pro-PTH. There are three forms of the circulating hormone: the biologically active complete hormone, 84 amino acids long, and biologically active amino-terminal fragments, each of which constitutes 10% of the circulating PTH – each with a half-life of ten minutes; the inactive carboxyl-terminal fragments make up the remainder of the PTH pool. PTH is a hypercalcaemic hormone and secretion is regulated by ionised calcium concentrations in the extracellular fluid. The effect is to modify renal vitamin D (1,25 dihydroxycholecalciferol) production to enhance calcium absorption from the gut mucosa. It also acts to increase distal tubal resorption in the kidney and release from bone to maintain serum calcium levels. Other preparations that promote vitamin D production include estrogen, prolactin, growth hormone and calcitonin. Calcitonin is a 32-amino-acid polypeptide, secreted from the C cells of the thyroid gland, which with its precursor katacalcin has a marked suppressor effect on calcium. It appears to act to modulate the effects of vitamin D and PTH in response to high serum calcium levels. The interleukin IL-1 has been shown *in vitro* to influence bone remodelling, which may also involve progesterone.

There are several conditions that influence bone calcium and therefore bone metabolism. Cushing syndrome with supraphysiological corticosteroid production will result in impaired osteoblastic skeletal formation and repair, decreased intestinal absorption and lower bone mass. Iatrogenic causes of loss of bone mass are seen with prednisolone and prolonged gonadotrophin-releasing hormone analogue treatment. Acromegaly resulting in growth hormone excess has an effect via somatomedins increasing bone growth but not bone mass. Thyrotoxicosis leads to excess bone turnover (associated with raised serum alkaline phosphatase, urinary hydroxyproline and deoxypiridinoline) and eventually osteoporosis, hypercalcaemia, reduced PTH and increased bone resorption. Estrogens and androgens have positive physiological effects on the skeleton and therefore also calcium metabolism.

---

**COMMON CAUSES OF HYPERCALCAEMIA**

- Malignancy
- Hyperparathyroidism
- Thyrotoxicosis
- Vitamin D poisoning
- Sarcoidosis

---

# Parathyroid hormone and calcium

Primary hyperparathyroidism was originally associated with osteitis fibrosa cystica but other presentations are more common.[2] Those less severe states can be screened for; 30% with raised PTH are asymptomatic. The prevalence is 1–3 in 1000, with an incidence of 25 per 100 000; it is twice as common in women as men. Excess PTH results in an exaggeration of its physiological effect and is due in 90% of patients to an isolated adenoma and in 2% as part of a multiple endocrine adenopathy (type 1 is associated with pituitary, parathyroid, pancreatic-islet and adrenal cortex lesions). In 5%, hyperparathyroidism is a result of hyperplasia associated with a strong family history of similar problems. A PTH-secreting carcinoma occurs in 1–2% of patients. Secondary hyperparathyroidism is associated with hypocalcaemia in renal failure and steatorrhoea. Iatrogenic causes for secondary hyperparathyroidism include lithium treatment and thiazide diuretic use. The bony abnormalities are marked in extreme cases, with increased bone resorption as a result of osteoclastic activity and osteoid deposition with osteoblastic activity. This results in disordered trabecular bone formation and a brittle structure with low bone mass. Cystic spaces within loose fibrous tissue that was occupied by marrow give the radiological appearances of osteitis fibrosa cystica and histological features of 'brown tumours of hyperparathyroidism'.

---

**CLINICAL PRESENTATIONS OF HYPERPARATHYROIDISM**

- Renal colic
- Bone pain
- Joint pain
- Lethargy, nausea, vomiting, weight loss,
- Constipation
- Polyuria, nocturia and polydipsia
- Psychiatric symptoms

---

Immunoradiometric assays demonstrate raised PTH levels and allow differentiation of hypercalcaemia (serum ionised calcium levels drawn from an arm with no tourniquet applied and corrected for serum albumin) with primary hyperparathyroidism from that associated with other causes with a normal or low PTH, e.g. malignancy. Supplementary investigations will demonstrate a low serum phosphate and raised serum alkaline phosphate in severe cases and urinary calcium and hydroxy-proline, elevated in proportion to alkaline phosphatase, reflecting simultaneous bone resorption and formation. Rarely a mild hyperchloraemic acidosis and aminoaciduria is seen.

Radiological tests demonstrate classical signs in 20% of patients. Subperiosteal erosions on the radial border of the middle finger, the ends of the clavicles, at the sacroiliac joint and at the symphysis pubis may be seen. Long-bone and skull cysts may also be seen. Bone mass is reduced and generalised osteopenia at cortical sites observed, e.g. the distal third of the forearm with lumbar sparing. Treatment reverses or stabilises these changes. Subtraction scintigraphy also has a role in localising abnormal parathyroid tissue.

Treatment is surgical for primary disease associated with bone, renal or psychiatric complications or if serum calcium persists beyond 2.25 mmol/l (corrected). In young asymptomatic patients, surgery may be necessary in those with impaired renal function (reduced creatinine clearance), hypercalciuria (greater than 400 mg/day) and significant osteoporosis in the distal radius. In less extreme cases, dietary advice, hydration, avoidance of diuretics and dietary calcium may suffice. In such cases, regular calcium assays, bone density and urinary calcium assessments should be made.

## Renal disease and calcium

The absorption of calcium is mediated by 1,25-dihydroxycholecalciferol (DHCC) by preferential resorption of calcium at the expense of phosphate in the kidney. 1-α-Hydroxylation of 25-hydroxy-vitamin D to form the active 1,25-DHCC is affected by renal disease, resulting in reduced production. An additional consequence is secondary hyperpara-thyroidism, which results in a combination of osteoporosis as well as osteomalacia. Osteomalacia is a failure of bone mineralisation resulting from vitamin D deficiency. In children with developing bones, this results in rickets; in adults, disordered bone remodelling results. Symptoms include long-bone pain, weakness (proximal myopathy without wasting), fatigue, and bow legs in children, with a characteristic waddling gait. The biochemical changes are lowered plasma calcium (partly corrected by hyperparathyroidism), lower plasma phosphate, raised alkaline phosphate, raised urinary hydroxyproline and normal plasma 1,25-DHCC (in renal tubular diseases such as Fanconi's syndrome, hypophosphat-aemic rickets and renal tubular acidosis). In renal failure, however, 1,25-DHCC is low. To differentiate dietary from renal causes of osteomalacia, serum levels that are normal point towards a renal cause but only a bone biopsy demonstrating widened osteoid seams and demineralised calcification fronts will confirm the diagnosis. Radiologically, bone demineralisation is focal, with the development of cysts or pseudo-fractures (Looser's zones) and vertebral bowing throughout the spine (unlike osteoporosis), resulting in a 'cod fish vertebrae', with normal bone density and a 'rickettsial rosary' in children. Treatment is vitamin D supplementation (1500–5000 iu/day), which results in a rapid initial recovery in muscle weakness but a concomitant temporary increase in bone pain. Bone healing takes several months and calcium with phosphate supplements are essential. In chronic renal failure, treatment initially requires 3 µg of calcitriol or 1 µg of alpha calcidol followed by a maintenance dose of 0.1 µg.

Hyperparathyroidism results in increased renal absorption of calcium and the formation of renal calculi. These present with renal colic two to three times more commonly than bone pain.

## Osteoporosis and calcium

This important condition affects an increasing proportion of women in their postmenopausal years, resulting in considerable morbidity. The clinical feature is an increased susceptibility to fracture as a result of a loss of bone mass, osteopenia, identified by low bone density on X-ray, and low scores for bone mineral content. The relationship between bone integrity and the estrogen family of steroids is well established. In the context of disordered calcium metabolism, osteoporosis represents a generalised skeletal disease with microarchitectural deterioration of bone tissue, bone fragility and susceptibility to fracture. Osteopenia represents the early stages of osteoporosis with a bone mass between 1 and 2.5 standard deviations below the mean for young adults, whereas osteoporosis represents a loss below 2.5 standard deviations of the young adult mean for age and sex.

Osteoporosis is usually secondary to systemic disease and only rarely presents as a primary disorder, namely juvenile, idiopathic, adult or senile osteoporosis. The disorders that lead to osteoporosis are hormonal, nutritional, renal, inflammatory, functional, neoplastic and, rarely, genetic (Table 17.1). Differential diagnoses include hyperparathyroidism, osteogenesis imperfecta and osteomalacia.

In men and women, there is a 3% loss in bone mass per decade after the age of 35 years. In women approaching their menopause, this accelerates to 9% until the age of 75 years and then returns to 3%. The skeleton is predominantly made of cortical bone. However, the burden of osteoporotic disease is borne by trabecular bone of the vertebral bodies, proximal femur, proximal humerus, distal forearm and pelvis. These are

**Table 17.1   Summary of the secondary causes of osteoporosis**

| Endocrine | Nutritional | Renal |
|---|---|---|
| Hypoestrogenism | Malabsorption | Bone disease |
| Vitamin D deficiency | Chronic hepatitis | |
| Cushing syndrome | Associated with osteomalacia | |
| Hyperthyroidism | Reactive hyperparathyroidis | |
| Hyperprolactinaemia | | |

**Table 17.1   A summary of the secondary causes of osteoporosis** (continued)

| Functional | Inflammatory | Neoplastic |
|---|---|---|
| Immobilisation | Chronic inflammatory bowel disease | Leukaemia |
| | Crohn's disease | |
| | Rheumatoid arthritis | |

the most common sites for age-related fracture with a lifetime risk of 39.7% in women. There is an increase in Colles' fracture from the age of 45 years and that of the vertebral body from 50 years onwards. Of the latter, only one in three will be symptomatic and consequently require relatively little medical input. Fracture of the neck of femur on the other hand has an incidence of 3% per year in women aged over 85 years, and represents a significant hospitalisation cost to the NHS. It gives a major contribution to mortality in this age group through indirect causes such as pneumonia and cardiac and cerebrovascular events.

Peak bone mass attainment is determined by genetic potential, nutritional, exercise-related factors and hormonal status. The regulation of bone mass and architectural development determines bone strength, which in turn determines fracture risk. The rate of loss of bone mass from a given initial density can be slow or rapid and thus remains difficult to predict. The density at any one time is, however, measurable and gives an indirect point assessment of bone strength.

The role of high dietary calcium intake in determining peak bone mass is now accepted. This is clearly demonstrated in studies of Japanese twins in whom one received dietary supplements and consequently achieved a higher bone mass.[3] In the UK, milk was the main dietary source of calcium in school-age children, until free supplies at schools were suspended. In estrogen-deprived women the average daily intake necessary to achieve neutral balance is 1500 mg per day compared with 1000 mg in premenopausal women. There is evidence that supplementing a calcium-poor diet can reduce bone loss and that this is potentiated by vitamin D supplements. In some ethnic racial groups, a high proportion lack intestinal lactase, which causes diarrhoea and steatorrhoea. Consequent avoidance of milk products accounts for poor dietary calcium absorption during adult life and an inadequate level for maintenance of bone integrity.

Calcium balance is also influenced by renal and other hormonal factors. Estrogen deficiency contributes to early development of osteoporosis in younger women with an early menopause and estrogen supplements in this group can help prevent loss of bone mass. This is reduced in obese women, whose circulating androstenedione is more readily converted to estrone peripherally. Weight-bearing and physical activity at all ages help maintain bone mineral content, with a minimum of three hours per week being necessary. Factors that counter calcium absorption include a high-protein diet. This is associated with acidic sulphur containing amino acids that promote urinary calcium loss. Foodstuffs or drinks high in phosphates and potassium promote calciuria. There is some evidence that fluoride supplementation of drinking water and moderate alcohol consumption can protect against a reduction in bone density loss.

Smoking has a deleterious effect but this may be due to an effect on ovarian function, resulting in earlier menopause and slimmer premorbid build, as any direct effect of smoking on calcium metabolism is unclear. Factors that confer some degree of protection against osteoporosis include obesity, through peripheral estrone production, increased dorsum-of-hand skin-fold thickness and black ethnic origin.

## References

1 Mundy GR, Oyajobi B, Traianedes K, Dallas S, Chen D. Cytokines and remodeling. In: Marcus R, Feldman D, Kelsy J, editors. *Osteoporosis.* 2nd ed. San Diego,CA: Academic Press; 2001. p. 373–404.

2 Woolf AD, Dixon A St J, editors. *Osteoporosis, A Clinical Guide.* 2nd ed. London: Martin Dunitz; 1998.

3 Johnston CC Jr, Miller JZ, Slemenda CW, Reister TK, Hui S, Christian JC, *et al*. Calcium supplementation and increases in bone mineral density in children. *N Engl J Med* 1992 Jul 9;**327**:82–7.

# Appendix
# Endocrine normal ranges

| | |
|---|---|
| Follicle-stimulating hormone | 2–8 iu/l (early follicular) |
| Luteinising hormone | 2–10 iu/l (early follicular) |
| Prolactin | < 500 mu/l |
| Thyroid-stimulating hormone | 0.5–5.0 iu/l |
| Thyroxine ($T_4$) | 50–150 nmol/l |
| Free $T_4$ | 9–22 pmol/l |
| Triiodothyronine ($T_3$) | 1.5–3.5 nmol/l |
| Free $T_3$ | 4.3–8.6 pmol/l |
| Thyroid-binding globulin | 7–17 mg/l |
| Testosterone | 0.5–3.5 nmol/l |
| Sex hormone-binding globulin (SHBG) | 16–120 nmol/l |
| Free androgen index ([testosterone x 100]/SHBG) | < 5 |
| Dihydrotestosterone | 0.3–1.0 nmol/ |
| Androstenedione | 2–10 nmol/l |
| Dehydroepiandrosterone sulphate | 3–10 µmol/l |

| | | |
|---|---|---|
| Cortisol | 8 a.m. | 140–700 nmol/l |
| | midnight | 0–140 nmol/l |
| | 24-hour urinary | < 400 nmol/24 hours |

| | |
|---|---|
| Estradiol | 250–500 pmol/l |
| Estrone | 400–600 pmol/l |
| Progesterone (midluteal) | > 25 nmol/l to indicate ovulation |
| 17-Hydroxyprogesterone | 1–20 nmol/l |

type 1  159
type 2  159
    hyperinsulinaemia and insulin
        resistance  168–9
    in PCOS  91, 105, 168
diabetic nephropathy, pregnancy and
    164, 166
diabetic retinopathy, pregnancy and
    164, 166
diclofenac  61, 62
diet
    calcium absorption and  195
    in diabetic pregnancy  164, 165
    lactating women  139–40
    see also nutrition
diethylstilbestrol-related uterine
    anomalies  11
dihydrotestosterone  197
1,25 dihydroxycholecalciferol (DHCC)
    190, 193
dilatation and curettage (D&C)  53, 57
dopamine agonists  140, 145–8
drugs
    affecting lactation  140
    affecting thyroid function tests  152
    inducing hyperprolactinaemia  143,
        145–6
dysfunctional uterine bleeding  55
dyslipidaemia, in PCOS  105–6
dysmenorrhoea  53, 73–5
    pathophysiology  54, 73
    primary  73, 74–5
    secondary  73–4, 75

eflornithine, topical  99
Endocell® endometrial sampler  57–8
endometrial ablation  67–70, 71
    efficacy and complications  69–70
    techniques  67–9
    vs hysterectomy  53, 70
endometrial aspiration (curettage)  57–8
endometrial assessment  57–9
    in amenorrhoea  80
    in PCOS  98, 111
endometrial biopsy  57–8
endometrial cancer
    after endometrial ablation  70
    detection  56–7
    endometrial hyperplasia risk  58

    in PCOS  98, 109–11
endometrial hyperplasia  56–7, 58, 59
    atypical  58
    in PCOS  98, 110, 111
    simple and complex  58
endometrial polyps  57, 59, 74
endometriosis, in müllerian duct
    anomalies  9, 12
epoöphoron  3, 4, 5
estradiol (E2)
    in menstrual cycle  47, 48–9
    serum  79, 197
estrogen(s)
    cardiovascular protection  185
    deficiency (hypoestrogenaemia)
        during lactation  139
        long-term sequelae  84, 87, 184–5
    in menstrual cycle  45, 47, 48–9
    plasma lipoproteins and  175, 176
    skeletal effects  191
    tumours producing  38–9
    uterine fibroids and  71–2
estrogen/progestogen therapy
    delayed puberty  43, 44
    menorrhagia  63, 64
    premature ovarian failure  185
    Turner syndrome  43, 182
    see also hormone replacement therapy;
        oral contraceptive pill, combined
estrogen therapy
    delayed puberty  44
    PCOS  99–100
    plasma lipoproteins and  176
    Turner syndrome  43, 182
    see also hormone replacement therapy
estrone  197
ethamsylate, for menorrhagia  61, 62
ethnic differences, plasma homocysteine
        in PCOS  106
exercise
    age at menarche and  34
    bone mass and  195
    in PCOS  96, 97, 106–7, 108, 119
    -related amenorrhoea  85–6
external genitalia
    ambiguous  5, 22, 23
    development  3–4, 5
    disorders of development  5–12
    examination  78

insulin sensitising agents
  in PCOS 97, 108–9, 124–6, 169
  in type 2 diabetes 168–9
interleukin 1 (IL-1) 191
intermediate-density lipoprotein (IDL)
  172, 174
intersex disorders 5–16
intracytoplasmic sperm injection (ICSI)
  129
intrauterine contraceptive devices 56
in vitro fertilisation (IVF)
  in PCOS 127–8
  in premature ovarian failure 186
in vitro maturation (IVM) of oocytes
  128–9
iodine 151, 152
  deficiency 154
  radioactive 156
iron deficiency anaemia, in menorrhagia
  55, 56, 59, 60
ischaemic heart disease (IHD)
  amenorrhoea and 80
  in PCOS 103, 107–8
  in postmenopausal women 175
  risk factors see cardiovascular risk
    factors

Kallman syndrome 43, 79, 115–16
Karman® endometrial sampler 57
karyotyping 79
ketoconazole 100

labia majora and minora, embryology
  3, 5
labioscrotal fusion 13, 22
labioscrotal swellings 5
lactase deficiency 195
lactation 137–42
  contraception and 140–1
  endocrine effects 139
  initiation 137
  maintenance, and milk letdown
    137–8
  metabolic effects 139–40
  pharmacological control 140
lactational amenorrhoea 139, 140–1
laparoscopic ovarian diathermy (LOD)
  123–4
laser endometrial ablation 68

LDL see low density lipoproteins
lecithin cholesterol acyltransferase 173,
  174
leiomyomas, uterine see fibroids, uterine
leptin
  amenorrhoea and 84
  in diabetic pregnancy 163
  in pubertal development 34–6, 41
letrozole, in anovulatory PCOS 121
leukotrienes, in dysmenorrhoea 54, 73,
  77
levonorgestrel intrauterine system (IUS),
  for menorrhagia 64, 71
LH see luteinising hormone
LHRH see gonadotrophin-releasing
  hormone
lifestyle modification, in PCOS 119–20
lipids 171–6
  dietary, transport 172–5
  endogenous transport 174
  hepatic metabolism 173–4
  plasma, postmenopausal women
    175–6
  see also dyslipidaemia
lipoprotein(a) 174, 176
lipoprotein lipase 172, 174, 175
lipoproteins 171–2
  transport 172–5
  see also specific lipoproteins
liver
  disease 82
  lipid metabolism 173–4
low density lipoproteins (LDL) 171,
  172–3, 174
  metabolism 174
  postmenopausal women 176
  receptors 172, 173, 174
luteinising hormone (LH)
  menstrual cycle 45, 46–7, 50
  pubertal development 29
  serum 197
    in amenorrhoea 79
    in clomifene-treated PCOS 120–1
    in PCOS 94–5, 118
luteinising hormone-releasing hormone
  (LHRH) see gonadotrophin-
  releasing hormone

macrosomia, fetal 166–7

thyroxine (T4) 151, 152
  free 152, 153, 197
  replacement therapy 155, 157
  total 153, 197
toxins, environmental 181–2
tranexamic acid, for menorrhagia 61,
    62, 65, 71
transcervical resection of endometrium
    (TCRE) 68
transforming growth factor (TGF) 48
transsphenoidal adenectomy 148
triglycerides 171–2
  serum 105, 175–6
  transport 172, 174
triiodothyronine (T3) 151, 152
  free 152, 197
  reverse (rT3) 152
  total 153, 197
troglitazone 109, 126
TSH see thyroid-stimulating hormone
tubal patency, assessment 115, 118
tumour necrosis factor 190
Turner syndrome 41–3, 182
  oocyte donation 186

ultrasound
  diabetic pregnancy monitoring 167
  endometrial assessment 98, 111
  in menstrual disorders 59, 72
  ovarian 95
  ovulation induction monitoring 121
  polycystic ovaries 91, 92, 93
urachus 5
urethral glands 5
urinary tract, developmental
    abnormalities 6
urogenital sinus 3, 5
uterine artery embolisation, for uterine
    fibroids 72–3
uterus
  anomalies 10–12
  arcuate 11
  bicornuate 11, 12
  development 3, 5
  didelphys 11
  diethylstilbestrol-related anomalies 11
  fibroids see fibroids, uterine
  perforation, endometrial ablation
    69–70

remnant (anlagen) 8
rudimentary horn 10–11, 12
septate 11, 12
unicornuate 10–11

Vabra® endometrial sampler 57, 58
vagina
  congenital absence (agenesis) 6–8
  development 3, 4, 5
  fusion abnormalities 8–10
  longitudinal septum 8
  transverse septum 9–10
vaginal dilators 7
vaginoplasty
  congenital adrenal hyperplasia 24
  McIndoe 7, 8
  tissue expansion 7
  Williams 8
vanillyl mandelic acid (VMA) 17, 18, 19
vascular endothelial growth factor
    (VEGF) 127–8
vasopressin, in dysmenorrhoea 73, 74
Vecchetti procedure 7
vertebral fractures 195
very-low-density lipoprotein (VLDL)
    171, 172, 173–4
vesicovaginal fistulae, after endometrial
    ablation 70
virilisation
  in congenital adrenal hyperplasia 13,
    22
  in precocious puberty 38, 39
visual field defects 87, 143
vitamin D 190, 193
  deficiency 193
VLDL see very-low-density lipoprotein
vomiting, in ovarian hyperstimulation
    syndrome 130, 131

waist circumference, in PCOS 96
waist-to-hip ratio 103, 105, 107, 119
weight, body
  lactating women 140
  loss, in PCOS 96, 97, 106–7, 108,
    119–20
  onset of puberty and 32–4
weight-related amenorrhoea 78, 83–4,
    116–17
Williams vaginoplasty 8